ALZHEIMER'S DISEASE AND RELATED CONDITIONS

A DEMENTOLOGIST'S HANDBOOK

First published in 1996. This edition first published in 2004.

ISBN 80 - 239 - 2529 - 6

Printed in Czech Republic by
MEDEA Press - M.Bransovsky, Rudolfov 373 71 - CZ

ALZHEIMER'S DISEASE AND RELATED CONDITIONS

A DEMENTOLOGIST'S HANDBOOK

Edited by

Antony Bayer
Jan Reban

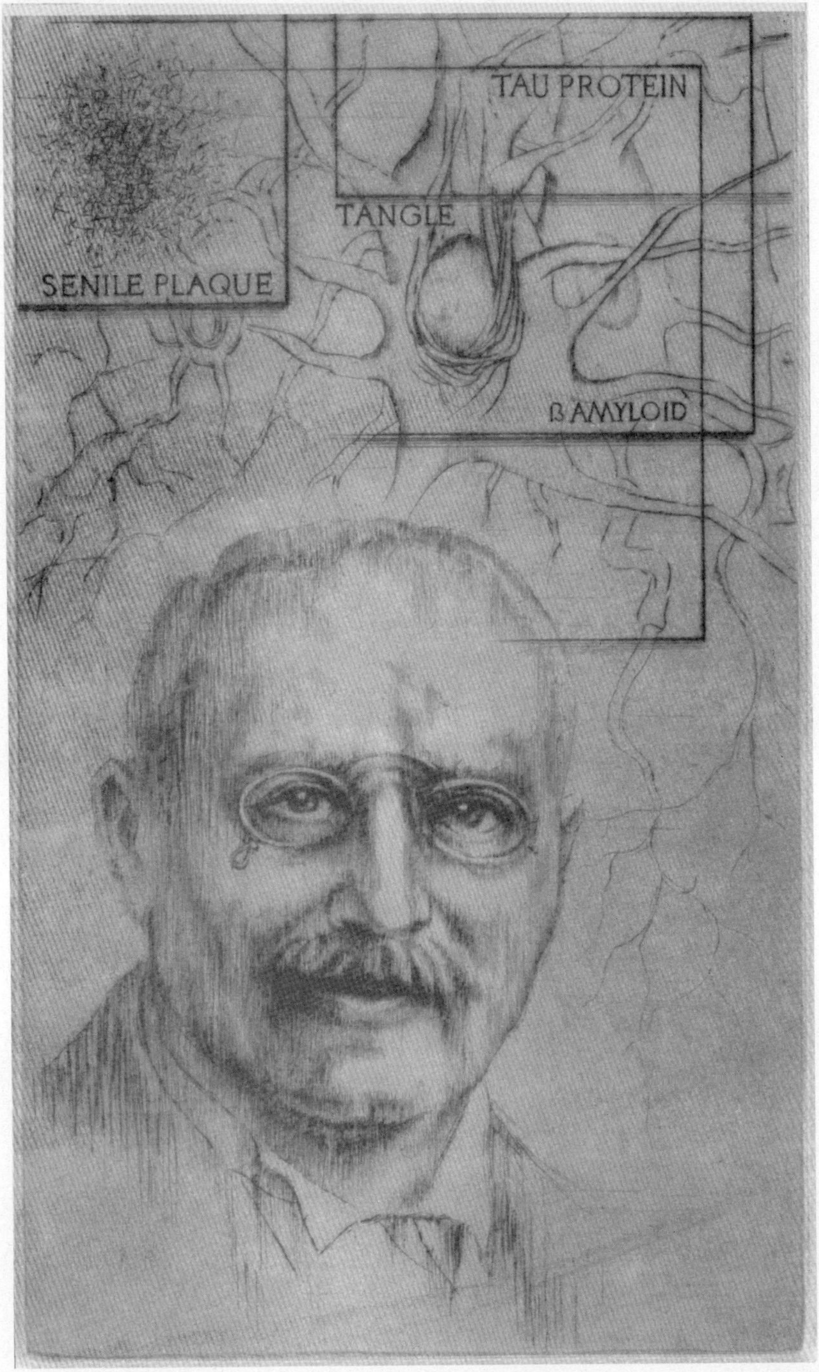

This bookplate , by the Czech artist Petr Minka , pays homage to Alois Alzheimer.
It is reproduced with artist´s permission.

CONTENTS

5. SPECIFIC PROBLEMS

APPENDICES

PREFACE TO THE FIRST EDITION

Over the years, the care of elderly and mentally ill people has shifted from institutions into the community and back again. But with each cycle some innovation and reform has been made.

Until the late 18th century, the mentally ill of any age were generally equated with criminals or beggars. It was Pinel who first coined the term 'demence' and introduced a model of disease and illness. Asylums created by him emphasised the benefits of active medical treatment and a positive environment. Under the influence of the Quakers in England, asylums became more open, and families were encouraged to visit their relatives. At the beginning of this century, the growing pressures of urbanization, industrialization and migration again made demands on institutions that increasingly became overcrowded. Just before the 2nd World War, the Marlborough Programme of Joshua Bierer drew attention to the potential of community-based care, developing social clubs for patients, day and night centers, after care and rehabilitation.

In recent years, the changing political map of Europe has provided both challenge and opportunity for the development of innovative approaches to care and closer collaboration and cross-national research. Inevitably different social, economic, cultural and environmental conditions will require alternative systems of management, but the issues and many of the solutions will be similar. The advantages of care within the community are widely acknowledged, but developments need to be fully evaluated before they are widely adopted. Emphasis should shift from merely considering structure and activity to carefully evaluating outcomes, not only in terms of morbidity and mortality, but also the overall benefit to quality of life and general wellbeing.

The importance of dementia as a major public health issue in all countries is now well recognized. Demographic changes suggest that the number of affected persons will continue to increase over the next few years and, by the year 2000, the European community will have in its midst some 6 million sufferers and perhaps up to 25 million family members with some degree of responsibility and personal involvement with their care. Most will be living outside institutions in their local community.

Professional intervention is likely to be most effective if it is interdisciplinary in approach, combining medical, psychological, nursing and social work expertise, with patients and carers assured of comprehensive assessment, management and support throughout the course of the illness. This model is the basis of the development of Community Memory Teams, which can provide optimal care through coordinated and informed interdisciplinary working. Cardiff's Memory Clinic was pioneering in this field and, with the support of the UN Trust Fund for Ageing, helped to develop the Community Memory Project in South Bohemia.

The objective of this Manual, prepared with collaboration of colleagues in the UK, Czech Republic, Austria, Slovakia, Japan and Spain, is to provide an overview of the important clinical aspects of assessment and management of dementing illnesses. It is hoped that this will serve as a useful initial reference for those setting up services for the demented, particularly in those European countries that are currently developing new approaches to the delivery of health and social care.

Antony Bayer, Cardiff / Jan Reban, Hluboka n/Vlt.
October, 1995

PREFACE TO THE SECOND EDITION

Any clinical or scientific publication soon becomes an antique, unless it is regularly refreshed. The field of dementia is rapidly evolving and, in the eight years since the first edition of this manual, there have been many changes in our understanding of Alzheimer's disease and other dementing conditions and in their management.

In 1996, the year when the first edition of this book appeared, van Gooi and van Grevel, writing in the Lancet, highlighted the fact that 1400 papers had been written on diagnosis and treatment of Alzheimer's disease in the previous 5 years. However, there appeared to be a discrepancy between the enthusiasm for the potential of this new knowledge and the conservation of traditional conservative methods in everyday practice. Fortunately the situation has begun to change in recent years. Clinical diagnosis is becoming more accurate and the importance of careful differential diagnosis to inform management is widely recognized. Promising developments from the fields of molecular biology, neurogenetics, neuroimaging and cerebrospinal biomarkers are helping to eliminate the word "probable" from definitions of dementias and removing the right of the pathologist to stamp the final diagnosis.

A decade ago, the possibility of effective drug treatments for the common dementias seemed a long time away, with the first clinical trials of the anticholinesterases just beginning to report. Now they have become the standard drug treatment for Alzheimer's disease, with emerging evidence of efficacy in vascular dementia, dementia with Lewy bodies and Parkinson's disease dementia. Already there are new approaches to treatment, based on modifications of amyloid and tau processing and use of stem cell and gene therapy technology. Developments in psycho-social management of dementia have also led to greater recognition of the patient as an individual, with strengths as well as weaknesses.

This rapid growth in clinical and research aspects of dementia encompasses many spheres of medicine and deserves recognition as a significant and independent specialty on its own. The emergence of the specialty of "Dementology" will help to resolve long running disputes over which specialty should take overall charge of assessment, diagnosis, treatment and care of this growing and increasingly demanding group of patients and their families. The dementologist will be ideally qualified to make decisions on best use of new technologies to aid diagnosis and on cost-effective prescription of the growing drug treatment options.

The title of the second edition of this book recognises the importance of the new specialty. Since the first edition, some new chapters have been added and all others have been updated and revised. We would wish to express our sincere appreciation to all the many colleagues who have made the publication of this book possible.

Jan Reban, Hluboka n/Vlt./ Antony Bayer, Cardiff.
January 2004.

EDITORS

Antony Bayer
Senior Lecturer in Geriatric Medicine
and
Director of the Memory Team,
University of Wales College of Medicine,
Llandough Hospital, Penarth CF64 2XX, Wales.
Email: bayer@cf.ac.uk

Jan Reban
University of South Bohemia , Health and Social Dept.
Center for Alzheimer´s Disease,
Geriatrician,GP
37341 Hluboka n/Vlt.,Masarykova 1, Czech Republic
Email: jreban@iol.cz

The book is dedicated to our families .

Eileen and children Rachel , Nick , Sam , Ben and Oliver
and
Vera and daughter Vera

ACKNOWLEDGEMENTS

The editors wish to express their appreciation to their colleagues who provided material for inclusion in this book: **Sergio Arino** *(Design and environment*), **Martin Bojar** *(Investigations*), **Donna Davies** *(Carer Support Groups),***Iva Holmerova** *(Czech Experience),***Victoria Diez-Rabago** *(Feeding and Swallowing),* **Eileen Flattery** *(Needs of carers),* **Mark Fish** *(Predementia and prevention),* **L.Glosova** *(Investigations),* **Malcolm Liddell** *(Sexual Problems),* **Gwen Phillips** *(Normal ageing - changes in brain function),* **Jennie Powell** *(Memory Albums, Communication problems, Feeding and Swallowing),* **Janice Rees** *(Cognitive Assessment - Principles and Approach, Driving),***Eva Sykova** *(Stem Cell Therapy),***Michael Syka** *(Neuroimaging),* **Christine Synan** *(Creative opportunities),* **Triona Rainsford** *(Individual Support for Carers,***Tami Tamitegama** (Sri Lanka Experience), **Jo Waring** *(Creative opportunities)* and to **Vladimir Vurm, Marion Kalousek**, **Vladimir Forst**, **Petr Petr** and **Stefan Krajcik** for help with its production.

We are also indebted to **Heather Copeland**, for her patience and perseverance in preparing the text for printing and to the **United Nations Trust Fund for Ageing** for their financial support of the first edition of this book.

For the help we must also thank to **Health and Social Dep. of South Bohemian University** and to pharmaceutical companies **Pfizer , Novartis , Janssen Cilag** and **Lundbeck** .

ABBREVIATIONS

AACD	Aging associated cognitive decline
AAMI	Age associated memory impairment
ACE	Angiotensin converting enzyme
ACE	Addenbrooke's Cognitive Examination
AD	Alzheimer's disease
ADAS-Cog	Alzheimer's Disease Assessment Scale – Cognitive Subscale
ADFACS	Alzheimer's Disease Functional Assessment and Change Scale
ADH	Antidiuretic hormone
ADL	Activities of daily living
AIDS	Acquired immune deficiency syndrome
AMT	Abbreviated Memory Test
APOE	Apolipoprotein E
APP	Amyloid precursor protein
BADLS	Bristol Activities of Daily Living Scale
BEHAVE-AD	Behavioural pathology in Alzheimer's disease Rating Scale
BSF	Benign senescent forgetfulness
CADASIL	Cerebral Autosomal Dominant Angiography with subcortical infarcts and leukoencephalopathy
CAMCOG	Cambridge Cognitive Examination
CAMDEX	Cambridge Mental Disorders of the Elderly Examination
CANTAB	Cambridge Neuropsychological Test Automated Battery
CAPE	Clifton Assessment Procedures for the Elderly
CAS	Caregiver Activity Survey
CDR	Clinical Dementia Rating
CDR	Cognitive Drug Research

CERAD	Consortium to Establish a Registry for Alzheimer's disease
CGI	Clinical Global Impression
CGIC	Clinical Global Impression of Change
CGIS	Clinician Global Impression of Severity
CIBIC	Clinician interview based impression of change
CIBIC-plus	Clinician interview based impression of change, plus carer interview
CDR	Clinical Dementia Rating
CBF	Cerebral blood flow
CBD	Corticobasal degeneration
CDQLP	Community Dementia QOL Profile
CIND	Cognitive impairment, not dementia
CJD	Creutzfeldt Jacob disease
CMAI	Cohen-Mansfield Agitation Inventory
CNS	Central nervous system
CSI	Caregiver Strain Index
CT	Computed tomography
DAD	Disabilty Assessment for Dementia
DCM	Dementia care mapping
DLB	Dementia with Lewy bodies
DQOL	Dementia Quality of Life Scale
DRS	Mattis Dementia Rating Scale
DSC MRI	Dynamic susceptibility contrast magnetic resonance imaging
DSM	Diagnostic and Statistical Manual of Mental Disorders
DWI	Diffusion weighted magnetic resonance imaging
ECG	Electrocardiogram
ECT	Electroconvulsive therapy
EEG	Electroencephalography
EMG	Electromyelography
ESR	Erythrocyte sedimentation ratio
fMRI	Functional magnetic resonance imaging
FPM	Functional Performance Measure

FTD	Frontotemporal dementia
GABA	Gamma aminobutyric acid
GDS	Geriatric Depression Scale
GDS	Global Deterioration Scale
GHQ	General Health Questionnaire
GMS	Geriatric Mental Schedule
HAROLD	Hemispheric asymmetry reduction in old adults
HIV	Human immunodeficiency virus
HVLT	Hopkins Verbal Learning Test
IADL	Instrumental activities of daily living
ICD	International Classification of Diseases
IDDD	Interview for Deterioration in Daily Living Activities in Dementia
IPA	International Psychogeriatric Association
VaD	Vascular dementia
MAOI	Monoamine oxidase inhibitor
MCI	Mild cognitive impairment
MI	Myoinositol
MMSE	Mini mental state examination
MRI	Magnetic resonance imaging
MRS	Magnetic resonance spectroscopy
MSU	Mid stream urine
NAA	N-acetyl aspartate
NINCDS-ADRDA	National Institute of Neurological and Communicative Disorders and Stroke – the Alzheimer's Disease and related Disorders Association
NINDS-AIREN	National Institute for Neurological Disorders and Stroke with support from the Association Internationale pour la recherché et l'Enseignement en Neurosciences
NMS	Neuroleptic malignant syndrome
NOSGER	Nurses Observation Scale for Geriatric patients
NPH	Normal Pressure Hydrocephalus
NPI	Neuropsychiatric Inventory

NSAID	Non-steroidal anti-inflammatory drug
NSF	National Service Framework
PD	Parkinson's disease
PDD	Parkinson's disease dementia
PDS	Progressive Deterioration Scale
PET	Positron emission tomography
PPA	Primary progressive aphasia
PS	Presenilin
PSP	Progressive supranuclear palsy
QOL	Quality of Life
QOL-AD	Quality of Life-AD Scale
RAGE	Rating Scale for Aggressive Behaviour in the Elderly
RCT	Randomised controlled trial
REM	Rapid eye movement
RISA	Radionucleide cisternography
RO	Reality orientation
SCB	Screen for Caregiver Burden
SEIQOL	Schedule for Evaluation of Individual Quality of Life
SIB	Severe Impairment Battery
SKT	Syndrom Kurztest
SLE	Systemic lupus erythematosis
SPECT	Single photon emission computed tomography
SSRI	Selective serotonin reuptake inhibitor
SNRI	Selective noradrenergic reuptake inhibitor
TIA	Transient ischaemic attack
WHO	World Health Organisation

1

BACKGROUND

1.1

HISTORICAL BACKGROUND

In the late 20th century, dementia (and Alzheimer's disease in particular) emerged from the shadows to be acknowledged as one of the most important medical conditions of the present day and the most significant cause of chronic disability and handicap in old age. Whilst only recently attracting the attention that it deserves, dementia has been recognised since ancient times.

Dementia in ancient times

- Early accounts of mental deterioration in old age were given by Ptah-Hotep (c. 3000BC) and can be found in the Ebers papyrus (c. 1550BC)

- In Greece, Pythagoras (c. 700BC) described the last stage of life as the 'senium', when 'the system returns to the imbecility of the first epoch of the infancy'. Hippocrates (c. 400BC) regarded mental decline in old age as inevitable, whilst Aristotle (c. 330BC) stated 'there is not much left of the acumen of the mind which helped in youth, nor of the faculties which served their intellect'.

- In Rome, Cicero (c. 200BC) wrote in De senectute that 'dotage' (senilis stultitia) was not typical of all older men, but only of those 'weak in mind and will.' He proposed that mental activity postponed 'senile debility', claiming 'intellectual activity gives buoyancy to the mind'. Aulus Cornelius Celsus first used the term 'demens' (without mind) in his book titled 'De re medicina' (c. 30AD).

- Galen (c. 200AD) recognised dementia ('morosis') as an illness of old age, describing 'some in whom the knowledge of letters and other arts are totally obliterated; indeed they cannot even remember their own names'.

Dementia before the nineteenth century

- With the fall of the Roman Empire, the Church became the most powerful influence on learning in the Western world and any disease or mental weakness was viewed as a punishment for sin. There was little empirical observation or thinking.

- Roger Bacon wrote the work 'Methods of Preventing the Appearance of Senility' in about 1260. He recognised the brain (rather than the heart) as the source of mental processes, but described old age as 'the home of forgetfulness' and 'senility as consequence of original sin'.

- In literature, Geoffrey Chaucer wrote in the Canterbury Tales 'with old folk, dotage is normal', whilst William Shakespeare gave many accounts of failing mental abilities in old age, most notably in King Lear and Hamlet. In his description of the seven ages of man in 'As You Like It', he refers to the 'last scene of all... is second childishness, and mere oblivion'.

- The first reference to the word 'demency' is by the English poet John Skelton, in 1522 and Richard Cosin, Vicar-General of Canterbury, used the word 'dementia' in 1592, when writing about insanity as a defence. He defined it as 'a passion of the mind, bereaving it of the light of understanding'.

- From the mid-1600s, medical textbooks were recognising various cognitive disorders, including memory loss. Thomas Willis, author of the 'Practice of Physick' wrote of 'stupidity, or morosis, or foolishness ... as a disease of the head or brain. Some at first crafty and ingenious become by degrees dull, and at length foolish by the mere declining of age'.

Table *Synonyms for dementia and Alzheimer's disease: from early times to the present day (based on Boller and Forbes 1998)*

- Alienation
- Amentia
- Anoea (extinction of imagination)
- Brainsickness
- Dotage or "second childhood"
- Fatuitat (silliness)
- Foolishness
- Idiocy
- Imbecility
- Insanity
- Lethargy
- Lunacy
- Madness
- Morosis
- Organic brain syndrome
- Phrenesis
- Presenile dementia
- Primary degenerative dementia
- Senile decay
- Senile dementia
- Senile psychosis
- Senility
- Simplicity
- Stupidity
- Witlessness

Dementia in the nineteenth century

- At the start of the 19th century in France, Phillippe Pinel coined the term '*demence*' to describe the condition where '*there is no judgement either true of false. The ideas appear to be insulated and to rise one after the other without connection*'. In his '*Treatise on Insan*ity' of 1806, he condemned the system of incarcerating the mentally ill in prisons and promoting the revolutionary idea that madness was a disease, not a crime.

- Pinel's student, Jean Etienne Esquirol, introduced precise terminology, defining dementia as '*the loss of mental faculties consequent on disease*'. This distinguished it from '*idiocy*' (learning disability), '*in which the intellectual faculties are never manifested.*' To underline the difference, he wrote, '*a man in a state of dementia is deprived of advantages which he formerly enjoyed; he is a rich man made poor. The idiot, on the contrary, has always been in a state of want and misery*'.

- Senile dementia became more narrowly defined, distinct from the then commonest cause of dementia, general paresis, and from '*dementia praecox*' (schizophrenia).

- Loss of brain weight accompanying dementia became increasingly recognised and in 1864, Thomas Wilks gave a definitive description of cerebral atrophy associated with alcoholism, neurosyphilis and senile dementia. It was widely believed that cerebral atrophy and senile dementia resulted from a gradual strangulation of blood supply to the brain, secondary to arteriosclerosis.

- In 1872, George Huntington wrote his paper '*On Chorea*', describing the symptoms of dementia characteristic of the condition that now bears his name. In 1894, Otto Binswanger published a paper on differential diagnosis of general progressive paralysis and described the condition of subcortical arteriosclerotic encephalopathy. In 1898, he also introduced the term pre-senile dementia. From 1892 to 1906, Arnold Pick described a series of cases of dementia associated with circumscribed atrophy of temporal and frontal lobes.

- By the last years of the century, improvements in microscopy, brain preservation and histochemical techniques had revolutionised the study of neuropathology.

The life of Alois Alzheimer

- Alois Alzheimer was born in Marktbriet am Main, near Wurzburg in central Germany, on June 14th, 1864. He studied medicine in Berlin, Tubingen and Wurzburg, writing his dissertation thesis on the histology of the ceruminal glands.

- On qualification in 1887 he first worked as an anatomy assistant, then as a carer for a woman with mental illness and then moved to become medical officer at the Municipal Mental Asylum (Hospital for the Mentally Ill and Epileptics) in Frankfurt am Main.

- During this time he published over 20 papers, mainly dealing with the histology of inflammatory and vascular brain diseases, including his description of 'arteriosclerotic brain atrophy' in 1895 and 'senile dementia' in 1898.

- In 1903 he moved to Heidelberg and then Munich as head of the Anatomical Laboratory at the Royal Psychiatric Hospital. His research colleagues included Franz Nissl, Frederick Lewy (who described the eponymous inclusion body found in PD and DLB) and Hans Creutzfeldt and Alfons Jakob (later to describe the spongiform encephalopathy which bears their name).

- On November 4th, 1906, Alzheimer presented the case of Auguste D, to the 37th Meeting of the South-West German Psychiatrists in Tubingen. The talk was titled 'About a peculiar disease process of the cerebral cortex' (Uber eine eigenartige Erkrankung der Hirnrinde'), but did not attract much interest from the audience. The full details were subsequently published, together with a description of a 56 year-old man called Johann F. who also suffered from dementia, associated with extensive plaque pathology, but no tangles.

- The Director of the Psychiatric Clinic in Munich was Emil Kraepelin, one of the founding fathers of biological psychiatry. In the 8th edition of his influential 'Handbook of

Psychiatry' published in 1910, he proposed the eponym of Alzheimer's disease, helping the condition to become accepted as a distinct clinical and pathological disease.

Alzheimer's first case

Auguste D was admitted to the Mental Asylum in Frankfurt am Main on November 25th, 1901. Aged 51 years, she presented with suspiciousness of her husband, rapidly increasing memory impairment and disorientation. She dragged objects here and there and hid them and at times believed that people were out to murder her and started to scream loudly.

Alzheimer's clinical evaluation largely consisted of simple psychometric testing, with questions systematically transcribed into her medical file notes along with the patient's answers. He asked about her name, her family, where she lived, the date and tested recent and remote memory, object naming, simple calculations, object recognition and reading and writing ability. A full medical examination was also completed. Over the next four and a half years, Auguste remained in the institution and in the last few months of her life, she developed sacral and trochanteric decubitus ulcers that led to septicaemia and pneumonia. Terminally she was described as 'totally dulled, lying in bed with legs drawn up and incontinent.'

After Auguste D's death on April 8th, 1906, Alzheimer examined her brain. This was described as 'consistently atrophic' and preparations stained with silver revealed 'peculiar changes of the neurofibrils, seen clustering together in thick bundles'. There were also 'miliary foci, distinguishable by the deposit in the cerebral cortex of a peculiar substance'.

Alzheimer seemed to have been especially interested by the early onset of the condition, its rapid progression and severity, its focal symptoms and the simultaneous presence of plaques and tangles. In the mid 1990s, the case notes of Auguste D and original histological sections were rediscovered.

- In 1912, Alzheimer accepted the chair of psychiatry in Breslau (now Wroclaw in Poland). Almost immediately he became ill with tonsillitis, accompanied by nephritis and arthritis and died of rheumatic heart disease on December 19th, 1915.

Developments in the 20th century

- After a slow start, scientific and clinical interest in dementia grew exponentially. With estimates suggesting the number of people with AD increased at least 20-fold in the 20th century, growing attention was given to the 'rising tide' and 'silent epidemic' of dementia. High profile sufferers of AD, such as Rita Hayworth, Ronald Reagan, Charles Bronson and Iris Murdoch caught the attention of the general public.

- In the 1960s, prospective clinico-pathological studies showed that senile dementia was predominantly due to AD. Distinction between pre-senile and senile dementia was seen as arbitrary, though special needs of those with early-onset dementia have been increasingly recognised.

- In the 1970s, the term 'subcortical dementia' came to describe the clinical picture of the dementia of Huntington's disease, progressive supranuclear palsy and some other degenerative and vascular dementias.

- In 1974, the concept of focal lesions resulting from strokes ('multi-infarct dementia') was proposed as the basis of most cases of vascular dementia. This replaced the longstanding notion of 'arteriosclerotic dementia' due to gradual strangulation of blood supply.

- In the 1980s, numerous reports detailed the pathological and clinical features of dementia with Lewy bodies (DLB) and it became recognised as the second commonest cause of degenerative dementia.

- Precise criteria for the diagnosis of dementia were first elaborated in the 3rd Edition of the Diagnostic and Statistical Manual of Mental Disorders of the American Psychiatric Association in 1980.

- The identification of the cholinergic deficit characteristic of AD (and DLB/PDD) led to clinical trials of potential drug treatments and the availability of anticholinesterase drugs.

- Developments in molecular biology identified beta amyloid derived from amyloid precursor protein as the main constituent of plaques in AD and Down's syndrome. The apolipoprotein E gene was implicated in sporadic disease and specific genetic mutations were demonstrated as responsible for the rare familial cases of AD. This allowed development of transgenic mouse models for research and new therapeutic approaches such as amyloid immunisation.

- Epidemiological studies identified numerous environmental and medical risk factors for dementia. Together with growing understanding of the role of inflammatory mechanisms, oxidative damage and inappropriate apoptosis underlying neuronal damage, this has opened the door to development of preventive treatment for the 21st century.

FURTHER READING AND REFERENCES

Alzheimer A. Uber eine eigenartige Erkrankung der Himrinde. Allg Zeitschr Psychiatr 1907; 64: 146-148. Translation in: Alzheimer Dis Assoc Disord 1987; 1: 7-8.

Berchtold NC, Cotman CW. Evolution in the conceptualization of dementia and Alzheimer's disease: Greco-Roman Period to the 1960s. Neurobiol Aging 1998; 19: 173-189.

Berrios GE, Freeman HL, eds. Alzheimer and the dementias. London: Royal Society of Medicine, 1991.

Devi G, Quitschke W. Alois Alzheimer, Neuroscientist (1864-1915). Alzheimer Dis Assoc Disord 1999; 13: 132-137

Graeber MB, Kosel S, Egensperger R, et al. Rediscovery of the case described by Alois Alzheimer in 1911; historical, histological and molecular genetic analysis. Neurogenetics 1997; 1:73-80.

Kraepelin E. Psychiatrie: Ein Lehrbuch fur Studierende und Arzte. Leipzig: Johann Ambrosius Barth 1910; 593-632. Translation in : Int J Aging Hum Dev 1985; 21: 235-238

O'Brien C. Auguste D and Alzheimer's disease. Science 1996; 273:28.

Plum F. Dementia: an approaching epidemic. Nature 1979; 279: 372-3.

1.2

NORMAL AGEING – *the older person in society*

The last century saw a revolution in public health, with improvements in nutrition, housing, education, health and social care. The transition from a state of high birth and death rates to one of low birth and death rates has resulted in a dramatic growth in the absolute and relative numbers of older people. Within one generation the proportion of the population aged over 80 years will double.

Informed analysis of the demography of ageing is essential for planning and formulating policies and programmes related to age-related conditions such as dementia.

The 'demographic revolution'

- In 1950, there were 205 million persons aged 60 years or over throughout the world. By 2000, the number had increased three-fold to 606 million and by 2050 it is estimated it will increase three-fold again, to almost 2 billion.

- Worldwide, I in 10 people is now aged 60+ years; by 2050, this will be 1 in 5 and by 2150, it will be 1 in 3.

- The older population itself is ageing, with the oldest old (80+ years) being the fastest growing segment of the older population. Over the next 50 years, the number of centenarians is projected to increase 15-fold, from the present 145,000 to 2.2 million. The biggest increase in numbers of centenarians will be seen in Japan, from less than 13,000 in 2000 to almost 1 million by 2050.

- A majority of older people are women (55%). Among the oldest old, the ratio of women to men is 2 to 1.

- Most countries in Northern and Western Europe currently have 13-18% of their total population aged 65+ years, whilst some Southern and Eastern European countries have yet to reach 10%. The countries with the lowest proportion of elderly people are now ageing fastest. In countries with already aged populations it is the proportion of the very elderly who are increasing

- In Europe, projected increases will be greatest in Eastern Europe, notably in Bulgaria, Romania, the Balkans and Poland.

- There are large continental differences; 1 in 5 Europeans are aged 60+, but only 1 in 20 Africans. The tempo of ageing in developing countries is faster than in developed countries and so they will have less time to adapt to the consequences of population ageing.

Table *World Population Ageing. Percentage of total population aged 60+ and 80+ years in 1950, 2000 and 2050, estimated by Economic and Social Affairs Department of United Nations, 2002.*

	Age 60 years or more			Age 80 years or more		
	1950	2000	2050	1950	2000	2050
Worldwide	8.2	10.0	21.1	0.5	1.1	4.1
United Kingdom	15.5	20.6	34.0	1.5	4.1	10.8
Czech Republic	12.4	18.4	40.1	1.0	2.3	9.5
Sri Lanka	7.3	9.3	27.6	0.9	0.8	5.4

The older person and society

In the past, the relatively small numbers of people surviving into old age were generally respected for their wisdom and experience and they often held positions of authority. Those in agricultural or domestic industries could continue to work for as long as they needed or wanted.

In contrast, in most of the modern world, old people tend to have low status and are regarded as contributing little to society, competing with the young, especially the unemployed, for state benefits and employment. The mass media tend to glorify youth and omit older persons or depict them in stereotypes. Globalization and the information technology revolution have largely sidelined older people, making existing imbalances all the more apparent.

In reality, most older people are active, independent and self-reliant and even more varied in their activities and interests that the rest of the population. It is therefore important not to generalise too much about 'the elderly' and to take care not to confuse the effects of illness with the effects of age. Effective health and social policy must be based on reality and potential, not stereotypes and myths.

Current demographic changes have major implications for contemporary society:

- an increase in prevalence of **age-related medical conditions**, such as dementia, stroke, ischaemic heart disease and osteoporosis. Whilst ageing is certainly not associated with inevitable disability and handicap, chronic illness becomes increasingly common in advanced old age and older people are liable to more domestic and other accidents.

- an increase in **expenditure on pensions and health care**. Often this is inadequate to meet the needs of an ageing population and elderly people are at greater risk of experiencing poverty, poor housing, isolation and avoidable morbidity

- an increase in the **burden of dependency** (a larger number of net consumers aged 65 years or older to be supported by taxes from a smaller number of economic producers aged 15-64 years; i.e. a change in the potential support ratio of pensioners to workers). Between 2000 and 2050, the dependency ratio will double in developed regions and triple in less developed regions.

- an increase in the **demand for social services provision**, particularly to look after older people living alone and without family support. The need for institutional care rises exponentially after middle age.

- an increase in **blurring of the boundaries of age**, as family, kinship and community structures change. Individual roles are no longer as tightly bound by chronological age, with growing numbers of older people regarding the "third age" to be an opportunity for new experiences and endeavours.

Table *Potential Support Ratio. The ratio of persons aged 15-64 years to those aged 65+ years in 1950, 2000 and 2050, estimated by Economic and Social Affairs Department of United Nations, 2002.*

	1950	2000	2050
Worldwide	**11.6**	**9.1**	**4.1**
United Kingdom	6.2	4.1	2.1
Czech Republic	8.2	5.0	1.6
Sri Lanka	10.0	10.8	2.9

Quality of life in old age

Long life alone is of doubtful value. It is the quality of life that makes life worth living at any age, providing a sense of purpose, individual expression, social interaction and good morale, even when physical or mental ability may be impaired.

The most important factors influencing quality of life of older people are:

- **Health.** Good health is universally desired, generally valued above any other attribute. Preventive care and active treatment of acute illness is appreciated in all circumstances, even in the presence of chronic disease. Maintenance of mental function is particularly treasured, with subjective complaints of forgetfulness independently correlating inversely with measures of global quality of life.

- **Loneliness** and isolation and lack of good interpersonal relations can rapidly lead to deterioration in quality of life. Maintenance of a well established social network of family, friends and neighbours is highly desirable and may help to reduce the incidence of dementia.

- **Income.** In many European countries, elderly people have an income that is too low to allow them to exist with comfort and confidence at home. The true value of state pensions is progressively falling.

- **Housing** problems largely relate to low income. Inadequate immediate environment increases dependency and vulnerability to falls, accidents, infection and hypothermia.

- **Terminal care**. Most older people would prefer to die at home, rather than in the impersonal surroundings of an institution. This should be possible if adequate support is available and distressing symptoms are appropriately treated. Older people deserve a good death as well as a good life.

It is a challenge to society to ensure that old age, regardless of disability, is a positive experience, a time of continuing satisfaction and purposefulness and a time when independence and self-determination are maintained for as long as possible.

FURTHER READING AND REFERENCES

Biggs S. Understanding Ageing. Milton Keynes: Open University Press, 1993.

Bond J, Coleman P, Pearce S (eds.) Ageing in Society: an Introduction to Social Gerontology (2nd Edition). London: Sage/Open University, 1993.

Jamieson A, Harper S, Victor C (eds.) Critical Approaches to Ageing and Later Life. Milton Keynes: Open University Press, 1997.

Johnson J, Slater R (eds). Ageing and Later Life. London :Sage Publications, 1993.

Tout K (ed). Elderly Care: A World Perspective. London: Chapman and Hall, 1993.

United Nations. Madrid Plan of Action on Ageing, 2002. (accessible at http://www.un.org/esa/socdev/ageing/waa/a-conf-197-9b.htm

Valliant GE. Aging Well. Boston: Little, Brown and Company 2002.

Vincent J. Politics, Power and Old Age. Milton Keynes: Open University Press, 1999.

1.3

NORMAL AGEING - *changes in the brain*

The structure and function of the brain change over the lifespan, with most change taking place in the very young and the old. The effects of normal ageing make elderly people more susceptible to the CNS effects of external factors, such as drugs and metabolic disturbance, and provide the baseline from which pathological states emerge. An understanding of the neuroanatomical and neurophysiological changes in the normal ageing brain is essential before interpreting a finding as abnormal.

- Age-related anatomical changes appear to be most marked in the prefrontal areas known to be associated with planning and executive function and in the temporal cortex, hippocampus and limbic system, known to be associated with memory and learning.

- Between the age of 20 and 90 years, brain weight declines by about 10% and ventricular size may increase 3 to 4 fold. Focal white matter abnormalities are seen in up to 80% of cognitively normal elderly subjects.

- Unlike cells in other organs, those in the central nervous system have limited ability to regenerate. However, several mechanisms mitigate age-related changes – **redundancy,** or **cognitive reserve** (i.e. initially more nerve cells than are needed), **plasticity** (i.e. new dendritic connections developing to make up for fewer cells) and **compensation**

(i.e. other areas of the brain taking over if one part is damaged)

- Age-related changes in the microscopic appearance of the brain include deposition of the pigment lipofuscin in nerve cells, deposition of amyloid in blood vessels and nerve cells and appearance of senile plaques and neurofibrillary tangles, similar to those seen to a much greater extent in AD.

- There is a gradual decrease in CBF and metabolism with advancing age, possibly related to decreased brain volume and atrophy. Lateralized patterns of brain activity tend to be less pronounced in ageing, a phenomenon described as hemispheric asymmetry reduction in old adults (HAROLD). CNS levels of neurotransmitters tend to fall, including dopamine, acetylcholine, serotonin, noradrenaline and GABA.

The clinical implications of these age-related changes are uncertain. Whilst conventionally it is thought intellectual function increases throughout childhood, peaks in early adult life and then declines, this model is too simplistic. Not all cognitive functions deteriorate with age and some may even improve. Memory abilities, executive skills and processing speed are especially vulnerable to ageing, but the extent of any decline is seldom dramatic enough to seriously affect the adaptive ability of most people.

General Intellectual Abilities

- With normal ageing there is some loss of **fluid intelligence** (skills associated with problem solving, novel tasks, new learning, speed of processing or inductive reasoning), but preservation of **crystallized intelligence** (use of previously acquired information and skills, general knowledge, comprehension and vocabulary).

- Studies of the Wechsler Adult Intelligence Scale indicate that verbal subtests remain relatively stable with ncreasing age, whereas scores on performance subtests (which rely mainly on non-verbal, visuo-spatial skills) decline. Though the performance subtests are timed and an age-related reduction in speed is therefore relevant, the discrepancy between the two scales remains even after the removal of time constraints.

- Verbal tests rely primarily on the use of previously stored information that is manipulated in familiar ways. Non-verbal performance tasks require the manipulation of novel material in unfamiliar and more complex ways. These tasks are more demanding and 'effortful' and a decline in ability would be consistent with older people having reduced processing resources.

Memory Functions

- Complaints about declining memory with advancing age are commonplace. Name finding and the 'tip-of-the-tongue' phenomenon are most common. However, self-report of memory impairment is more highly correlated with depression scores than with performance on memory tests.

- Memory is a very complex construct and many different models have been conceived to provide explanations of its many facets.

    - **Primary Memory.** This relates to immediate recall, for example holding briefly a telephone number whilst it is dialled. There is a little evidence this changes with normal ageing.

    - **Secondary Memory.** To remember information in primary memory for longer than a few seconds requires rehearsal so that it can be retrieved after a short time rather than immediately. This secondary memory does show an age related decline. Thus it has been demonstrated that older subjects are less likely to spontaneously utilise organisational and semantic encoding strategies and make less efficient use of rehearsal strategies. Age differences are more noticeable on tasks requiring free recall than on tasks of cued recall or recognition. Self initiated retrieval processes that are voluntary, intentional and effortful become increasingly more difficult to execute with advancing age.

- **Working Memory** The need to carry out further operations while holding information stored in secondary memory has been referred to as working memory. Tasks such as mental arithmetic and backwards digit span involve a component of divided attention, requiring the holding of information in an active state whilst carrying out the mental operation. This makes demands on the pool of processing resources and older people are more vulnerable than younger to interference in tasks involving divided attention.

- **Tertiary Memory.** Ability to recall memories from the past that are firmly held in the memory store, such as general knowledge and childhood memories, does not seem to change much with age. Claims that remote memory improves with age are unsubstantiated.

- Overall, older subjects perform less well on tasks requiring unaided recall and losses in source and contextual memory (where and when an event took place). Primary memory, recognition memory, memory for general knowledge and vocabulary and procedural memory (e.g. playing the piano) decline little.

Capacity for New Learning

- Studies have traditionally focused on age related deficits in new learning capacity. This is especially so for non-critical material and new languages. There is now a belief that new skills can be acquired in late life and there is greater reserve capacity and potential for new learning than previously thought. Appropriate training may need to be more intensive.

Speed of Reaction

- Both central ('decision making') and peripheral ('motor') components of reaction time slow with age and age-associated differences increase with the complexity of the task (i.e. choice reaction time deteriorates faster than performance on a simple reaction time task). However, inter-individual differences are much more significant than any effect of age.

Individual differences

- As age increases, so does the variability between and within individuals. 'Average performance' becomes less representative of individuals. Many studies have shown that factors such as poor health, low education and lower intelligence produce a greater effect on cognitive performance than chronological age.

- There is also growing evidence suggesting an interaction between memory and participation in leisure activities. Keeping oneself busy and stimulated might have a beneficial effect on cognitive function in the later life.

FURTHER READING AND REFERENCES

Craik FIM, Salthouse TA, Mahwah NJ (eds). The Handbook of Aging and Cognition. New Jersey: Lawrence Erlbaum Associates, 1999.

Cullum S, Huppert FA, McGee M, et al. Decline across different domains of cognitive function in in normal ageing. Int J Geriatr Psychiatry 2000; 15: 853-862.

Grady CL, Craik FIM. Changes in memory processing with age. Current Opinion in Neurobiology 2000; 10: 224-231.

Rabbitt P, Lowe C. Patterns of cognitive ageing. Psychological Research 2000; 63: 308-316.

Small S, Stern Y, Tang M, et al. Selective decline in memory function among healthy elderly Neurology 1999; 52:1392-6.

Stuart-Hamilton I. The Psychology of Ageing. London: Jessica Kingsley, 1991.

1.4

EPIDEMIOLOGY OF DEMENTIA

The ageing of the world's population means that the number of people with age-related conditions such as dementia will inevitably increase.

Across the world, 25 million people are estimated to have dementia and perhaps up to 100 million family members and carers with some degree of responsibility and personal involvement with the sufferers. In Europe, there are about 8-10 million people afflicted with dementia and 1.5 million new patients every year.

Estimating numbers of people who have dementia is not easy.

- There are particular problems of definition (e.g. distinguishing mild dementia from age-related cognitive change and agreeing criteria for ante-mortem diagnosis of AD and VaD)

- Care must be taken to ensure the exclusion of patients with poor mental performance due to other conditions (e.g.acute confusion, low intelligence, lack of education, hearing and visual impairment and depression).

- Study populations must be carefully chosen, taking care to avoid referral bias and that the very elderly and those in institutions are not under represented.

- Recent identification of biomarkers in cerebrospinal fluid, developments in the field of molecular biology and advances in neuroimaging has potential for improving the clinical diagnosis of dementia.

Most recent epidemiological studies have used a two stage approach to identification - an initial screening test, such as the mini mental status examination, to first identify those with normal mental function, followed by more intensive assessment of the remaining subjects using standardised interview schedules, such as the CAMDEX or GMS/AGECAT.

Prevalence And Incidence of Dementia

- Prevalence data (an estimate of the proportion of people with dementia within a population at any one time) are valuable for planning services and particularly for assessing the extent of unmet need and for generating hypotheses about possible causes.

- Incidence rate (an estimate of the number of people developing dementia over a specified time period) is not affected by survival rates and allows the predictive validity of aetiological hypotheses to be tested. However, the necessary cohort studies are time consuming, costly and difficult to carry out.

- The overall prevalence of dementia after age 65 is about 5-10% and the annual incidence is 1-2%. After age 75 the prevalence is 15-20% and the incidence about 2-4%. In people under the age of 60 years, dementia is seen relatively rarely, with a prevalence of about 0.08%.

- Both prevalence and incidence rates rise exponentially with age, with a doubling around every 5 years over the age of 60. There is little evidence to suggest levelling off in extreme old age. More than 85% of dementia cases occur in those aged over 70 years.

- The lifetime risk of becoming demented (assuming a normal lifespan) is about 1 in 4. There is no current evidence to suggest that incidence rates are changing.

In the United States, AD ties with stroke as the third most common cause of death.

- Age-adjusted prevalence rates for Alzheimer's disease are higher for females than males, whilst for vascular dementia the converse is possibly true.

Table *Estimated prevalence (%) of dementia by age and gender (adapted from Ott et al, BMJ 1995; 310: 970-973)*

Age Group (years)	Estimated prevalence (%)		
	Men	Women	Both sexes
55-59	0.2	0.6	0.4
60-64	0.5	0.4	0.4
65-69	0.8	1.0	0.9
70-74	2.0	2.1	2.1
75-79	6.0	6.2	6.1
80-84	13.7	19.3	17.6
85-89	28.4	32.7	31.7
90+	41.2	40.6	40.7
All 65+	5.9	11.5	9.4
All 75+	13.2	20.2	18.1

- Recent studies in China and South East Asia suggest lower prevalence rates than in European studies; dementia prevalence in those aged 65+ years was 1.8% in Singapore and 1.7% in Taiwan. In Bangkok it was 7.5%. These differences may be attributable to regional differences in risk factors, or may merely reflect variations in methodology.

- The average yearly cost of care for people with dementia in the USA is estimated to be $35,287 per patient, generating an annual cost to the US economy of more about $150 billion.

FURTHER READING AND REFERENCES

Fratiglioni L, Launer LJ, Andersen K, et al. Incidence of dementia and major subtypes in Europe: a collaborative study of population-based cohorts. Neurology 2000; 54 (suppl 5): S10-S15.

Hofman A, Rocca WA, Brayne C, et al. The prevalence of dementia in Europe: a collaborative study of 1980-1990 findings. Int J Epidemiol 1991; 20: 736-48.

Jorm AF. The Epidemiology of Alzheimer's disease and related disorders. London: Chapman and Hall, 1990.

Jorm AF, Jolley D. The incidence of dementia: a meta-analysis. Neurology 1998; 51: 728-33.

Kukull WA, Bowen JD. Dementia epidemiology. Med Clin North Am. 2002;86:573-90.

Lobo A, Launer LJ, Fratiglioni L, et al. Prevalence of dementia and major subtypes in Europe: a collaborative study of population-based cohorts. Neurology 2000; 54 (suppl 5): S4-S9.

Mayeux R. Epidemiology of neurodegeneration. Annu Rev Neurosci 2003; 26: 81-104.

Prince M. Dementia in developing countries. A consensus statement from the 10/66 Dementia Research Group. Int J Geriatr Psychiatry. 2000;15:14-20.

Roman GC. Vascular domentia may be the most common form of dementia in the elderly. J Neurol Sci. 2002;15;203-204:7-10.

Sadik K, Wilcock G. The increasing burden of Alzheimer disease. Alzheimer Dis Assoc Disord. 2003;17 Suppl 3:S75-9.

Wimo A, Winblad B, Aguero-Torres H, et al. The magnitude of dementia occurrence in the world. Alzheimer Dis Assoc Disord. 2003;17:63-7.

Winblad B, Wimo A, Mobious H-J, et al. Severe dementia: a common condition entailing high costs at individual and societal levels. Int J Psychiatry 1999; 14: 911-4

1.5

PRE-DEMENTIA AND EARLY DETECTION

Complaints about declining memory with advancing age are commonplace. Differential diagnosis is essential to distinguish an unnecessary concern about the insignificant changes that normally accompany ageing, from the many important conditions that may have complaints of poor memory as part of their presentation.

Identifying people who are likely to progress to dementia whilst they are still relatively asymptomatic will help to ensure that interventions to slow or prevent progression can be targeted on those most in need. Effective identification of predementia states and timely intervention will have a substantial benefit to individuals, their families and society.

There is a confusing plethora of inconsistently used terminology, with only some criteria reliably identifying a pre-dementia syndrome.

Benign senescent forgetfulness (BSF)

- BSF was a term coined in 1962 by the Canadian clinician, Vincent Kral, to distinguish memory problems in residents of a nursing home that were benign from those that were malignant (fulfilling present dementia criteria) and associated with poor prognosis.
- The hallmarks of the condition were an awareness of problems, inability to recall incidental details from the

recent past rather than whole events and the 'tip of the tongue phenomenon', with recall some time later. Importantly there had to be no clinical evidence of memory dysfunction (though no specific tests were specified). However, Kral acknowledged that minor memory lapses might be a harbinger of malignant forgetfulness (i.e. dementia) in some cases.

Age associated memory impairment (AAMI)

- AAMI was proposed by a National Institute of Mental Health Work Group in 1986. It refers to persons aged 50 years and older who are experiencing a decline or loss in memory function reflected in everyday life and who perform at least one standard deviation below the mean of younger people on standardized tests of recent memory. The person must be otherwise healthy, with adequate intellectual function and without delirium, depression or dementia, determined by a MMSE score of greater than 23. Vast numbers of elderly people meet these criteria and only a minority will progress to dementia.

- Important points about this designation are the use of a statistical cut off with the comparator being young adults, the requirement for both subjective memory complaints and an objective measure, and the specification of memory as the cognitive domain of interest.

- Problems include its over-inclusiveness and the lack of specification of standardized cognitive test (depending upon which test or tests are used between 7 and 96% of healthy elderly may meet the criterion) and its use of a cross-sectional measure with a population-based cut-off to describe individual decline.

- This term should probably not be used as a clinical diagnosis unless the aim is to pathologise the majority of elderly people. This is not a pre-dementia syndrome, with the estimated 1% annual dementia incidence similar to that of the general age-matched population.

Aging-associated cognitive decline (AACD)

- An International Psychogeriatric Association and World Health Organization Working Party proposed the designation of AACD in 1994. Although sounding similar to AAMI, it is distinct in many important respects. Subjective complaint *or* informant report of cognitive decline is necessary and difficulties can occur in *any* one of the following cognitive domains: memory, attention/concentration, abstraction, language and visuo-spatial function. Performance on cognitive testing must be one standard deviation below the mean for an *age and education-matched* population. Evidence of systemic, psychiatric or neurological disorder is an exclusion criterion and decline must have been evident for at least 6 months. As with AAMI, onset must be gradual and dementia is not present

- This designation identifies individuals who are doing badly in relation to their peers on cognitive tests, but does not imply any defined pathological process. Individuals with sudden onset of problems or those with no insight and no reliable informant would not meet the criterion. Although this is not implied by its title, this is another cross-sectional measure.

Mild cognitive disorder (MCD)

- MCD was included in the tenth edition of the International Classification of Diseases to describe documented cognitive decline associated with systemic or central nervous system disease, which it does not outlast by more than a few weeks, and not so severe as to fulfill criteria for dementia. Memory or concentration may be affected and there is usually an objective cognitive deficit. It is distinct from delirium.

- **Mild neurocognitive disorder** is a similar DSM IV diagnostic category that requires a significant degree of functional impairment, and includes substance abuse as a cause.

Mild cognitive impairment (MCI)

- MCI refers to complaints of memory loss in elderly people that are considered to have a high probability of evolving into dementia. It is explicitly construed as a 'transitional zone between normal aging and very probable Alzheimer's disease.' As in AAMI, memory is the specified cognitive domain. Like AACD, comparison is made with age and education matched peers.

Table *Clinical criteria for MCI.*

1. A self-reported memory complaint, preferably corroborated by a family member 2. A detectable memory deficit abnormal for age and education (about 1.5 SD or more below the norm) 3. Normal general cognitive function aside from memory 4. Ability to carry out such activities as driving a car and balancing a cheque book 5. Absence of dementia

- Studies suggest that MCI and AD have similar anatomical localisation, with the main difference being functional rather than structural, and in severity of impairment.

- About 10% of the population aged 65 years or more may fulfil criteria for MCI and longitudinal studies indicate 10-15% of people these will progress to dementia each year, compared with a rate of 1-2% in control subjects.

- MCI is a very useful diagnosis in clinical settings to apply to patients who present with memory complaints, but is less useful in epidemiological studies or screening programmes where subjects with no complaints and with a range of cognitive deficits may be encountered. Those without insight do not meet the criterion.

- Proposals have been made to alter the core definition and criterion of MCI to capture the prodromes of dementia types other than AD, such as 'vascular cognitive impairment' where multiple domains of cognition or a single non-memory domain may be affected. It is recommended for clarity's sake that the term MCI is qualified with an appropriate modifier such as *amnesic* MCI, because MCI has often been used as a term for cognitive impairment in general, rather than the specific diagnostic condition.

Cognitive Impairment, No Dementia (CIND)

- CIND is an umbrella term that includes AACD and MCI within its scope. It is applied to cases where there is an objectively defined cognitive impairment, but insufficient evidence to warrant a dementia diagnosis. Often when it is applied, reference is made to age and education matched norms.

- As CIND makes no presumptions about aetiology or progression, it includes a heterogeneous group of patients and so, without qualification, it is not very helpful in a clinical context. However, the lack of restrictive criteria can be useful in epidemiological studies, as the term can be applied to subjects doing poorly on cognitive tests but not clearly fitting into any other category. Patterns of cognitive deficit can be investigated without pre-conception - memory impairment is not a necessary component. A disadvantage may be that there is more variation in the application of the term between studies.

- A recently explored designation is ‘vascular cognitive impairment, no dementia’, or 'vascular CIND'. This is applied where there is objective cognitive impairment and clinically significant vascular features on assessment, yet failure to meet the functional threshold for dementia. It identifies subjects who are at greater risk of institutionalization than non-vascular CIND subjects.

Early Detection Of Cognitive Decline And Dementia

Early detection is essential for implementing strategies to reverse or prevent further cognitive decline and to plan future management. A number of approaches to early detection are available:

- **Neuropsychological assessment.** This is clearly the most practical approach as it measures directly the function of interest. However, it can be time-consuming and the considerable inter-individual variation in cognitive abilities and age-related cognitive decline may make it difficult to interpret a single neuropsychological assessment, even using age and education-related norms. Serial measurement is more valuable, though even a single assessment can identify an individual's strengths and weaknesses and be used to guide intervention tailored to the individual. Brief screening tests, such as the MMSE, will detect more severe cognitive impairment and most cases of established dementia, but are insensitive to early dementia. Computer-based technology may be useful for both evaluation and training.

- **Neuroimaging**. Structural and functional neuroimaging can detect the early changes in the brain that develop before the clinical expression of MCI or dementia. Measurement of hippocampal atrophy by MRI and metabolic changes in the temporoparietal cortex by PET have shown most promise, but are expensive and not widely available for population use. Recent developments allow the imaging of amyloid deposits in the brain, that may be useful for detecting preclinical AD and for measuring progression after therapeutic intervention.

- **Biomarkers.** Early detection of AD has investigated use of CSF levels of beta amyloid and tau protein and blood levels of beta amyloid. Genetic markers include the susceptibility apoE4 gene for AD, though this is not associated with increased risk of cognitive decline with ageing. Future genetic profiling, combined with neuropsychological and neuroimaging measures may help to identify high risk populations for targeted intervention.

FURTHER READING AND REFERENCES

Crook T, Bartus RT, Ferrris SH, et al. Age Associated Memory Impairment: proposed diagnostic criteria and measures of clinical change. Report of a National Institute of Mental Health Work Group. Dev Neuropsychol 1986; 2: 261-76.

Hogan DB, McKeith IG. Of MCI and dementia: improving diagnosis and treatment. Neurology 2001; 56: 1131-2

Kral VA Senescent Forgetfulness: Benign and Malignant. Can Med Assoc J 1962; 86: 257-60.

Levy R. Aging Associated Cognitive Decline. Int Psychogeriatr. 1994; 6: 63-8

Morris JC, Storandt M, Miller JP, et al. Mild cognitive impairment represents early-stage Alzheimer's disease. Arch Neurol 2001; 58: 397-405.

Palmer K, Wang H-X, Backman L, et al. Differential Evolution of Cognitive Impairment in Nondemented Older Persons: Results from the Kungsholmen Project. Am J Psychiatry 2002; 159: 436-442

Petersen RC, Doody R, Kurtz A, et al. Current Concepts in Mild Cognitive Impairment. Archives of Neurology 2001; 58: 1985-1992

Petersen RC, Stevens JC, Ganguli M, et al. Practice parameters: early detection of dementia: mild cognitive impairment (an evidence based review). Neurology 2001; 56: 1133-43.

Ritchie K, Artero S, Touchon J. Classification criteria for mild cognitive impairment. A population-based validation study. Neurology 2001; 56: 37-42

Tuokko H, Frerichs RJ. Cognitive Impairment with No Dementia (CIND) Longitudinal Studies, the Findings, and the Issues. Clin Neuropsychol 2000; 14: 504-525

1.6

PREVENTION OF DEMENTIA

The prevention of dementia has enormous potential benefits for the individual, their families and for society as a whole. Some of the factors associated with increased risk of developing dementia may be influenced by attention to lifestyle, vascular risk factors and active management of other medical conditions, as well as through pharmacological interventions

Lifestyle factors

- Low education and poor linguistic ability in early adult life and social disengagement in late life are independent risk factors for cognitive decline and dementia. Definitive evidence from prospective, randomized controlled trials is not available, but maintaining social and family activities, keeping mentally active and possibly formal memory training (the 'use it or lose it' argument) would all seem to be valuable preventive interventions, perhaps by promoting biological 'cognitive reserve'.

- Continued complex occupational or voluntary work challenges individuals to communicate and participate in exchanges that stimulate cognition and may promote increased synaptic complexity and neurogenesis.

- Chronic stress can lead to hippocampal atrophy and may reduce 'cognitive reserve'. Strategies to reduce stress may therefore help to preserve cognitive function.

- Physical exercise improves cognitive function in animals, possibly through increasing neurotrophins. Regular aerobic exercise in older people is associated with maintenance of cognitive function, but the direction of the association is not certain and any beneficial effect may be mediated indirectly by improved mood, reduction in stress or improved vascular risk.

- A balanced healthy diet is likely to help cognition. Malnutrition and isolated vitamin deficiencies can cause long-term cognitive impairment. Antioxidant vitamins may be important in protecting the brain against damage from oxidative stress and some studies suggest that a diet rich in vitamin E and C is protective against dementia. Other studies have suggested benefits from regular fish consumption, a diet high in monounsaturated fats and a light to moderate alcohol consumption.

Controlling vascular risk factors

Older people with a high burden of vascular risk factors are at 2 to 3 fold increased risk of developing dementia, suggesting that treatment of hypertension, hyperglycaemia and hyperlipdaemia and thromboprophylaxis for atrial fibrillation might reduce risk.

- Risk of developing dementia is reduced if BP is controlled in mid-life. In the Syst-Eur trial, treating isolated systolic BP in people over 60 years halved the incidence of dementia.

- Hyperlipidaemia is associated with cerebral atrophy and increase in beta amyloid deposition in the brain. Cross-sectional studies suggest use of statin drugs is associated with up to 70% lower risk of developing dementia. However, the apparent benefits of statins may be related to mechanisms other than lowering blood cholesterol. Prospective RCTs are in progress.

- Diabetes mellitus in mid-life is a risk factor for cognitive decline and improved control of blood sugar is associated with improved cognitive function. The benefit of tight glucose control on incidence of dementia is uncertain.

- Anticoagulation for chronic atrial fibrillation greatly reduces risk of stroke and is therefore likely to reduce cognitive impairment. Primary prevention of vascular cognitive decline with low dose aspirin is logical, but there is no supportive RCT evidence.

Managing other medical conditions

- Depression is the commonest reversible cause of cognitive impairment in older people. People with a high sense of self-efficacy are more likely to maintain cognitive function over time and past history of major depression is a risk factor for dementia.

- Sleep fragmentation, sleep apnoea and chronic use of sedative drugs may adversely affect learning and concentration abilities. Promotion of sleep hygiene and avoidance of daytime naps may improve quality of nighttime sleep.

- Both prescribed and over the counter medications should be used wisely. People with reduced cognitive reserve will be at especial risk of central nervous system side effects of drugs.

- Hearing and visual deficits can be a cause of social isolation, loss of mental stimulation and low mood and their treatment may help to maintain cognitive function.

- Smoking is associated with increased vascular disease, but probably not with AD. Nicotine may enhance attention, but overall is likely to be detrimental to long term cognitive ability.

- Long term heavy alcohol consumption is associated with dementia. Abstinence may halt or reverse cognitive decline. Long term marijuana abuse is probably associated with subtle deficits in memory, concentration and information processing, though the severity of impairment is much less than with alcohol abuse.

Table. *Strategies to prevent cognitive decline and dementia (adapted from Fillit and Butler, 1997).*

Lifestyle management

- Build cognitive reserve by remaining intellectually and socially active
  - Continue lifelong learning ('train the brain')
  - Engage in regular mental exercise ('use it or lose it')
  - Maintain active social networks
  - Remain involved in the community by occupational, religious or voluntary activity
- Engage in regular physical exercise
- Reduce or minimize the effects of stress
- Ensure appropriate nutrition and avoid nutritional deficiencies
- Light to moderate alcohol consumption

Medical management

- Hypertension
- Diabetes
- Hyperlipidaemia
- Depression
- Sleep disorders
- Polypharamacy
- Sensory impairments
- Avoid excess alcohol, smoking and illicit drugs

Pharmacological management

- Cognitive enhancers
- Neurotrophins
- Anti-inflammatory drugs
- Antioxidants
- Hormones

Pharmacololgical management

At present there is no proven drug treatment that will prevent cognitive decline or delay the progression of MCI to dementia.

- Recently a large trial of combined oestrogen/progesterone treatment to prevent development of AD was stopped early when risk of dementia (and stroke) was found to be greater in patients on active treatment than placebo. This was contrary to evidence from epidemiological studies and emphasizes the importance of only relying on evidence from well-designed prospective RCTs.

- Preliminary data suggest that cholinesterase inhibitors may improve cognitive ability in some people with MCI, though benefit is small and progression to AD does not seem to be prevented. RCTs of glutamate modulators and ampakines in MCI and for prevention of cognitive decline are ongoing. Huperzine, phosphatidylserine and gingko biloba are promoted to enhance cognitive ability and prevent decline, but with little supportive evidence of efficacy in RCTs. Other drugs being investigated in RCTs include neurotrophins, NSAIDs, statins, antioxidants, testosterone in hypogonadal men and dehydroepiandrosterone.

- Treatments that reverse or stabilize the deposition of amyloid, such as immunotherapy and secretase inhibitors, may have a more fundamental influence on the development and course of Alzheimer's disease.

FURTHER READING AND REFERENCES

Fillit HM, Butler RN. Cognitive decline: Strategies for Prevention. London, Greenwich Medical Media, 1997.

Gorelick PB, Erkinjuntti T, Hofman A, et al. Prevention of vascular dementia. Alz Dis Assoc Disord 1999; 13: S131-9

Sherwin B. Mild cognitive impairment: potential pharmacological treatment options. JAGS 2000; 48: 431-441.

Small SA. Age-related memory decline: current concepts and future directions. Arch Neurol 2001; 58: 360-4.

1.7

DIFFERENTIAL DIAGNOSIS OF DEMENTIA

Complaints of poor memory or signs of confusion are all too often assumed to indicate dementia, without sufficient effort to determine their true nature or a precise diagnosis. Because such a wide variety of conditions can provoke or mimic a confusional state, careful differential diagnosis is an essential first step in management.

Important issues to remember when considering differential diagnosis are:

- Age-related changes in memory are of greater concern to some patients than to others and must be distinguished from a pathological condition of prognostic significance.
- The commonest cause of a true confusional state in elderly people is delirium not dementia
- Depression is the most prevalent mental disorder of old age.
- Drug-induced confusion is commonly overlooked but easily reversed once identified.
- Deafness and focal cortical deficits of dysphasia or dyspraxia may present as an apparent memory problem or dementia.
- Many patients will have more than one factor contributing to their problems.

Delirium

An acute confusional state may develop in patients with previously normal mental state. However, it is most common in those whose brain function is already compromised, for example by pre-existing dementia.

Characteristically it is of relatively abrupt onset and brief duration and characterised by fluctuating disturbance of attention, cognition, behaviour and wakefulness.

Most cases of delirium will rapidly and completely resolve with appropriate treatment. Nevertheless, compared to control patients, those with delirum have both longer hospital stays and increased mortality and a minority may have long- term cognitive sequelae.

Table *Causes of delirium*

***Physical causes*:**
- infection (intracranial and extracranial)
- cardio-respiratory disease
- metabolic disturbance and dehydration
- acute stroke or transient ischaemic attack
- trauma
- post-epilepsy
- urinary retention
- constipation
- hypothermia
- drug intoxication or withdrawal (including alcohol)

Sensory causes:
- pain, poor vision and hearing

Psychological causes:
- anxiety, stress, paranoid states

Environmental causes:
- sensory deprivation or overload
- unfamiliar environment

Differentiation of delirium from dementia is usually straightforward if a careful history is obtained, ideally from a close relative or neighbour.

Table *Characteristic features of delirium and dementia*

Delirium	***Dementia***
Acute (over hours or days), with relatively sudden onset	Chronic (over months or years) with insidious or stuttering onset
Usually reversible	Usually irreversible
Fluctuating conscious level and alertness	Fully conscious and normally alert
Short attention span, easily distracted	Attention span less obviously changed and may perseverate
Disorganised thinking	Impoverished thinking
Apathetic, often delusional	Fearful
Variability of cognitive state from hour to hour, often worse at night	More consistent cognitive and behavioural change
Accompanying physiological changes	Physiologically stable

Drugs

Prescribed and over the counter drugs are the commonest cause of reversible confusion in adults. The ageing brain has less cognitive reserve and is therefore especially sensitive to this effect, perhaps by a factor of two to three.

Psychoactive medication and anticholinergics are the usual cause, but any drug with central nervous system activity may be implicated. Symptoms generally respond rapidly to drug withdrawal or dose reduction.

Table *Drugs causing or exacerbating confusion in older patients*

Psychotropics
Barbiturates
Benzodiazepines
Butyrophenones
Chlormethiazole
Hypnotics
Phenothiazines

Antidepressants
Lithium
MAOIs
Tricyclics
Trazodone

Anti-Parkinsonian
Amantadine
Anticholinergics
Dopamine agonists
Levodopa
Selegiline

Anticonvulsants
Carbamazepine
Gabapentin
Lamotrigine
Phenytoin
Sodium valproate
Vigabatrin

Anticholinergics
Anti-parkinsonians
Atropine
Oxybutynin
Propantheline
Scopolamine (transdermal)

Antihistamines
Diphenhydramine
Promethazine
Chlorpheniramine

Antimicrobials
Acyclovir
Cephalosporins
Chloramphenicol
Chloroquine
Ciprofloxacin
Gentamicin
Isoniazid
Rifampicin
Sulphonamides

Analgesics
NSAIDs
Narcotics
Tramadol

Cardiovascular
Beta-blockers
Clonidine
Digoxin
Diuretics
Methyldopa

Other
Aminophylline
Baclofen
Caffeine
Cimetidine
Corticosteroids
Doxapram
Hypoglycaemics
Interferon
Prochlorperazine
Theophylline

Drug withdrawal
Alcohol
Barbiturates
Benzodiazepines
Chlormethiazole
SSRIs

Depression

Major depressive illness presenting with the clinical picture of dementia has been termed 'psudodementia'. The diagnosis is perhaps most often established with hindsight.

Table *Features helping to distinguish depression and dementia*

Depression	*Dementia*
Fairly abrupt onset and duration in weeks	Insidious onset and duration in months or years
Constant low mood and sadness, associated anxiety	Fluctuating mood, still able to be happy
Answers questions with 'don't know' or refusals	Guesses answers and 'near misses'
Relatively intact sense of time and direction	Disorientation occurs early
Improvement with practice; absence of rapid forgetting	Little improvement with practice and rapid forgetting
Volunteers failings; highlights subjective difficulties	Denies or conceals failings in recall
Variable cognitive performance	More consistent cognitive performance
Memory loss develops after depression	Depression may develop after memory loss
Associated sleep, libido and appetite disturbance	Sleep, libido and appetite initially unchanged
Previous/family history of depression	Family history of dementia of depression

Subjective memory complaint may be a prominent feature of depression in older people, especially in the 'young old'. Severe depression may be associated with objective cognitive impairment, particularly on complex tasks and timed tests.

About 20% of those presenting to memory clinics will have a primary depressive disorder underlying their symptoms. Any suspicion of depression in a patient who also appears to be dementing is a justification for antidepressant treatment.

FURTHER READING AND REFERENCES

Arie T. Pseudodementia. Br Med J 1983; 286: 1301-2.

Blazer DG. Depression in Late Life, 3rd edition. New York, Springer Verlag, 2002.

Chiu F (ed). Functional Psychiatric Disorders. Cambridge, Cambridge University Press, 1994.

Gray SL, Lai KV, Larson EB. Drug-induced cognition disorders in the elderly: incidence, prevention and management. Drug Safety 1999; 21: 101-122.

Lavretsky, H., Kumar, A. Clinically significant non-major depression: old concepts, new insights. Am J Geriatr Psychiatry 2002, 10: 239-55.

Lindesay J, Rockwood K, MacDonald A. Delirium in Old Age. Oxford: Oxford University Press, 2002.

Lipowski ZJ. Delirium: Acute Confusional States. New York: Oxford University Press, 1990.

Visser, P.J., Verhey, F.R., Ponds, R.W., Kester, A., Jolles, J. Distinction between preclinical Alzheimer's disease and depression. J Am Geriatr Soc 2000, 48: 479-84.

Wells CE. Pseudodementia. Am J Psychiatry 1979;136:895-900

Yousef, G., Ryan, W.J., Lambert, T., Pitt, B., Kellett, J. A preliminary report: a new scale to identify the pseudodementia syndrome. Int J Geriatr Psychiatry 1998, 13: 389-99.

2

THE DEMENTIAS

2.1

ALZHEIMER'S DISEASE

Alzheimer's disease (AD) is the commonest cause of dementia, responsible for about half of all cases in autopsy series. A diagnosis of definite AD can only be made when histopathology is available and so in life, most patients can only be identified as having probable (or possible) AD. Standard diagnostic criteria (the McKhann or NINCDS-ADRDA criteria) have been widely adopted and correctly identify 80-90% of cases.

Formerly AD was used only for people with young onset dementia, but the distinction between 'presenile' and 'senile' dementia is now recognised to be spurious and the term AD is applied to both. Although incidence is very closely related to age, AD is not an inevitable part of ageing. There appear to be distinct clinical and pathological differences between people with early AD and those with age-related cognitive changes.

Risk Factors

As well as old age, other confirmed risk factors for AD are:

- a history of dementia in first-degree relatives, especially in early onset cases. In a very small proportion of patients, the condition shows autosomal dominant transmission, with identified mutations on chromosome 21 (in the APP gene), the presenilin-1 (PS-1) gene on chromosome 14 and PS-2 gene on chromosome 1. Over 70 mutations capable of producing the clinical and pathological features of AD have so far been identified on these three genes, 60 of them on the PS-1 gene.

- Specific genetic polymorphisms increase risk of developing AD. The best established is the e4 allele of the ApoE (apolipoproteinE) gene on chromosome 19. Normally present in about 12% of the population, it is found in 40% of people with AD (at expense of the e3 allele which is reduced in frequency). Heterozygotes carry 3 times and homozygotes 8 times the risk of developing the disease. It appears to affect primarily the age of onset of the disease.

Table. *Apolipoprotein E genotype, age of onset of AD and estimated effect on life expectancy (adapted from Warwick Daw et al, Am J Hum Genet 2000; 66: 196-204).*

	Apolipoprotein E genotype				
	e4/e4	e3/e4	e2/e4	e3/e3	e2/e3
Mean age at onset of AD (years)	71.2	75.2	77.3	81.2	89.4
Change in life expectancy (SE) (years)*	-6.4	-2.4	-0.3	+3.6	+11.8

** based on mean age of onset of AD in population*

- Down's syndrome in the subject (and possibly in a first degree relative).
- a history of atherosclerotic disease and associated factors (hypertension, hypercholesterolaemia, homocysteinaemia, ischaemic heart disease, stroke and diabetes mellitus)

Other possible risk factors for developing AD include late maternal and young paternal age at time of the subject's birth, female sex, western rather than eastern nationality, lack of education, history of previous head trauma, depression, sleep apnoea or hypothyroidism and family history of Parkinson's disease. Recent studies suggest that lifestyle characterized by engagement in leisure activities of an intellectual and social nature is associated with slower cognitive decline in healthy elderly people and may reduce the risk of AD.

The use of statin drugs or NSAIDs have been reported to have a potential protective effect in epidemiological studies and results from prospective RCTs are awaited. Contrary to epidemiological evidence suggesting that oestrogen therapy may be associated with delayed onset and reduced risk of developing AD, a recent RCT showed an increased incidence of dementia. Similarly, whilst early studies suggested a protective effect of smoking, recent larger studies show that persistent cigarette smoking does not reduce (and may increase) age-specific incidence of AD.

Table. *Possible risk factors for Alzheimer's disease*

Confirmed	Possible
Old age	Female sex
Family history of dementia	Family history of PD
Atherosclerotic disease	Western nationality
ApoE e4	Advanced maternal age
Down's syndrome	Cigarette smoking
	Low education
	Homocyseinaemia
	Diabetes mellitus
	History of hoad injury
	History of depression
	History of sleep apnoea
	History of thyroid disease
	History of lymphoma
	Lack of physical activity
	Lack of intellectual activity
	Poor social network
	Statin drugs (protective)
	NSAIDs (protective)
	Herpes simplex infection
	Exposure to aluminium
	Solvent abuse

Pathology

- The typical neuropathological features of AD are neuritic plaques (containing beta amyloid) and neurofibrillary tangles (paired helical filaments of hyperphosphorylated tau protein). Confirmation of the diagnosis relies on quantitative (e.g. plaque count) rather than qualitative features. Both plaque and tangle count correlate with dementia severity, although the best correlation is with the degree of synaptic loss.

- Other histopathological features of AD include dystrophic neurons, granulovacuolar degeneration, congophilic angiopathy and Hirano bodies. The distribution of the changes is characteristic, with the limbic and paralimbic systems and associated cortex most and the motor and calcarine cortex least affected.

- Much recent interest has centred on the role of beta amyloid in AD. This is the main constituent of the core of the neuritic plaque and is formed from amyloid precursor protein (APP). Mutations within the APP gene are responsible for some cases of early onset, dominantly inherited AD. Transgenic mouse models with this mutation develop Alzheimer's plaque (but not tangle) histology, which can be prevented by immunisation with beta amyloid 42. The APP gene is over-expressed in Down's syndrome (where AD changes inevitably develop). Beta amyloid deposition also occurs after head injury and may be increased in the presence of APOE-e4.

- APP is normally processed by an alpha secretase pathway, that results in a soluble end product that cannot form plaques, or a beta and gamma secretase pathway that produces both 40- and 42-amino acid beta amyloid peptides. The amyloid deposited in neuritic plaques is predominantly the 42-amino acid form, which has a greater potential to aggregate than the more common 40-amino acid peptide. In AD, intraneuronal accumulation of
- 42-amino acid beta amyloid is thought to increase phosphorylation of tau,

leading to the formation of neurofibrillary tangles, whilst extracellular accumulation leads to neuronal dysfunction and cell death. This in turn precipitates micoglial activation and an inflammatory response that further compromises brain function.

Clinical Features

- The earliest symptom of AD noticed by patients and their families is usually the insidious onset of forgetfulness and inattention. Other presenting cognitive deficits may include impairment of language, visuo-spatial skills, problem solving, abstract reasoning and judgement. Sometimes the initial symptom is of personality, behaviour or mood change.

- Initially, short-term memory and new learning are especially affected, with little material entering long-term storage and therefore able to be retained. Subsequently, immediate and remote memory are progressively lost. Recognition is in general less impaired than free recall and inconsistent retrieval over-repeated test trials and a greater -than-normal number of false positive responses is characteristic.

- Mild word-finding disturbance is often apparent from an early stage. Younger patients seem to have greater problems with language than the very old. Speech progressively becomes more circumlocutory and lacking in content, and comprehension becomes impaired. In late stages, language is limited in both quality and quantity and the patient may become mute.

- Spatial and perceptual problems may manifest as problems recognising familiar places or faces, or difficulties carrying out activities such as getting dressed, setting the table, or making a hot drink.

- Characteristically patients are less aware and concerned about their problems than those around them and this loss of insight often means they are not greatly distressed by their condition.

Symptoms progressively worse, usually over 5 to 10 years, but there is great variability in rate of decline and some patients, especially the very old, seem to remain stable for years. With increasing loss of social skills and deterioration in personal habits, the patient becomes totally dependent. Death is usually due to seticaemia from pneumonia, urinary tract infection or pressure sores.

Diagnosis

- Without histopathological confirmation, the diagnosis of AD depends on excluding other causes of dementia and identifying clinical features (especially pattern of neuropsychological deficits) that are characteristic.

- CT and MRI may confirm atrophy (especially of the medial temporal lobe and hippocampus) and serial assessment is especially useful. SPECT/PET scans may show characteristic bilateral temporo-parietal deficits.

- The EEG is likely to show generalised slowing, but is not useful diagnostically. The measurement of CSF beta amyloid and tau protein can aid diagnosis, but is not used routinely.

- Serial cognitive assessment is helpful to document progression.

- Assessment of APOE status is not recommended, as it is neither necessary nor specific for the diagnosis in any individual patient. Genetic testing for specific mutations may be indicated in younger people with a strong family history and after appropriate counselling.

Use of the NINCDS-ADRDA criteria will improve clinical diagnosis, with over 80% sensitivity and specificity.

Management

Whilst there remains no specific therapy that has been proven to influence the course of AD, the introduction of anticholinesterase drugs for mild to moderate disease and memantine for moderate to severe disease has had a major impact on symptomatic management. Specific symptoms may also benefit from drug treatment, particularly anti-depressants for mood disorders, hypnotics for sleep disturbance and neuroleptics for psychotic symptoms and agitation.

Active medical management of concurrent medical conditions, planning and design of the patient's living environment, psychological therapies and support, timely referral to new services to match changing problems, attention to the needs of family carers and active management of terminal care will all help to enhance patients' quality of life.

FURTHER READING AND REFERENCES

Bianchetti A, Trabucch M. Clinical aspects of Alzheimer's disease.Aging (Milano). 2001;13:221-30.

Burns A, Howard R, Pettit W. Alzheimer's Disease : a Medical Companion. London, Blackwell Science, 1995.

Clark CM, Karlawish JHT. Alzheimer disease. Current concepts and emerging diagnostic and therapeutic strategies. Ann Intern Med 2003; 138: 400-410.

Gauthier S. Clinical diagnosis and management of Alzheimer's disease.(2nd edition) London, Martin Dunitz, 1999.

Grossberg GT. Diagnosis and treatment of Alzheimer's disease. J Clin Psychiatry. 2003;64 Suppl 9:3-6.

Hofman A, Ott A, Breteler MM, et al. Atherosclerosis, apolipoprotein E and prevalence of dementia and Alzheimer's disease in the Rotterdam Study. Lancet 1997; 349: 151-4.

Lim A, Tsuang D, Kukull WA, et al. Clinico-neuropathological correlation of Alzheimer's disease in a community-based case series. J Am Geriatr Soc 1999; 47: 564-9.

Seshadri S, Drachman DA, Lippa CF. Apolipoprotein E4 allele and the lifetime risk of Alzheimer's disease – what physicians know, and what they should know. Arch Neurol 1995; 52: 1074-9.

2.2

DEMENTIA WITH LEWY BODIES AND PARKINSON'S DISEASE DEMENTIA

There is a spectrum of syndromes associated with the pathological finding of Lewy bodies. The clinical picture is related to their distribution and concentration within different brain regions.

When dementia dominates (often with prominent neuropsychiatric features) and accompanies or precedes the development of Parkinsonism, the condition has been variously named the Lewy body variant of Alzheimer's disease, Lewy body dementia, or diffuse or cortical Lewy body disease. It is now generally known by the consensus title of dementia with Lewy bodies (DLB) and is recognised as the second most common cause of degenerative dementia, after AD.

When Parkinson's disease (PD) precedes the development of dementia by at least 12 months (24 months in some definitions), the condition is termed Parkinson's disease dementia (PDD). The distinction between DLB and PDD does not seem to have a clear biological basis, but is widely used clinically.

Pathology

- Lewy Bodies are intraneuronal eosinophilic inclusion bodies, the detection of which has been made easier by using immunocytochemical staining with an antibody to ubiquitin. They are thought to result from a failed attempt by neurones to dispose of abnormal proteins. After binding to ubiquitin, the proteins accumulate within the Lewy body in the nerve cell, rather than being subsequently broken down by proteolytic enzymes.

- In PD, Lewy bodies characteristically are found localised in the brain stem nuclei. In patients with PDD and in DLB they are more widely distributed through the deeper layers of the neocortex and parahippocampus. They are rare in the hippocampus.

- The severity of dementia correlates with the density of neocortical Lewy Bodies, which are often associated with senile plaques. These are diffuse, unlike the neuritic plaques of AD. There is also accompanying diffuse neuronal cell loss, but neurofibrillary tangle formation is less consistently found.

- DLB and PDD are associated with atrophy of the nucleus basalis of Meynert and loss of cholinergic innervation of the cortex. Cholinergic deficits in DLB are more severe than in AD. Dopaminergic deficits are also more severe in DLB than AD, and in PDD than PD without dementia.

DEMENTIA WITH LEWY BODIES

Epidemiology

- Autopsy results from hospital-based series have reported prevalence of DLB between 17 to 36% of all dementia cases, though in unselected community series the prevalence is 11 to 22%. The condition may be slightly more common in men.

- There is sometimes a family history of PD and/or AD. The alpha-synuclein gene on chromosome 4 and the CYP2D6 gene have been implicated in a few cases. The APOE-e4 is more frequent in DLB than in nondemented PD or control patients and common genetic risk factors may explain the overlap of DLB and AD pathology.

The average rate of decline in DLB is slightly faster than in AD, with a mean duration of illness of about 5-7 years. However, the course can be very variable.

Clinical features

DLB is characterised by the clinical syndrome of fluctuating dementia, motor signs of parkinsonism and neuropsychiatric features, notably visual hallucinations. The consensus criteria for diagnosis of probable DLB have high specificity but limited sensitivity.

- **Cognitive impairment** is the initial symptom in two thirds of cases and characteristically fluctuates in severity (over hours or weeks). This is associated with varying levels of alertness and lucidity, much as is seen with delirium. Relatives may complain that the patient seems to switch off for periods of time and lacks concentration. There is a variable performance in ability to carry out daily living activities. The development is insidious and progressive

- **Parkinsonism** is often present at presentation and may predate cognitive impairment, though usually only by a few months. Unlike in classic PD, rigidity and bradykinesia are more often symmetrical, resting tremor is unusual, myoclonus may be present and response to levodopa is not dramatic and may be absent. Some patients with findings typical of DLB at autopsy show no extrapyramidal features during life.

- **Neuropsychiatric symptoms** develop in about 80% of DLB patients and occur earlier in the course of the illness than in AD. They most commonly take the form of persistent, detailed and stereotyped visual hallucinations, often of people or animals or unusual objects around the home. They tend to be most problematic at night and may recur over many months. Many patients seem to be able to recognise them as unreal. There may be associated delusional symptoms, often paranoid, misidentifications and less commonly hallucinations in other domains.. Other behavioural problems such as agitation and wandering are unusual, at least before the late stages of the illness. Depression is a possible supportive feature.

- **Unexplained loss of consciousness** (often mistaken for TIA or fits, but without focal neurological signs or other corroborative evidence) and repeated falls also support the diagnosis. Rapid eye movement (REM) sleep behaviour disorder (characterised by vivid dreams and their acting out whilst asleep), nocturnal periodic limb movements and excess daytime sleepiness are more common than with other dementias.

- **Sensitivity to neuroleptic drugs** is characteristic, occurring in up to half of DLB patients. Even very small doses may lead to severe extrapyramidal signs in patients without previous Parkinsonism. In extreme cases this may take the form of the neuroleptic malignancy syndrome (NMS), consisting of marked muscle rigidity and akinesia, pyrexia, autonomic failure and lowered conscious level. This has an associated mortality of up to 25% and should be regarded as a medical emergency.

The overall profile of DLB tends to differ between clinical settings. In psychiatric clinics, the condition generally will be seen as a dementia with prominent hallucinations and delusions; in medical out patient settings it is more likely to present as a Parkinsonian syndrome with dementia; on acute hospital wards it may be mistaken for delirium and only recognised when patients are found to be particularly sensitive to neuroleptic drugs.

Assessment

There are no clinical measures that will specifically identify DLB, but the presentation should suggest the diagnosis. The sensitivity and specificity of the consensus clinical criteria in prospective autopsy-validated studies are 0.83 and 0.95 respectively. The main differential diagnosis will be from AD, VD, PDD and PD-plus syndromes.

- On cognitive testing in early DLB, patients often perform especially poorly on measures of executive function, attention, problem solving, verbal fluency and visuo-spatial skills and relatively better on tests of verbal and logical memory. Repeated cognitive testing may document fluctuating ability.

- Neuroimaging may show generalised cortical atrophy, or may be entirely normal. Medial temporal lobe and hippocampal volume is less diminished than in AD, but more than in controls. Compared to AD patients, SPECT scans in pure DLB show less parieto-temporal and more occipital hypoperfusion. The main value of imaging will be to exclude other pathology, especially stroke disease.

- The EEG in DLB may show early slowing of background activity and excessive fluctuation of frequency from second to second, but this is of little value in diagnosis of individual patients.

Management

- Advantage can be taken of lucid periods to explain and discuss the nature of the problems and to build on retained abilities. Involvement of physiotherapy, occupational therapy and speech therapy is helpful.

- Anti-Parkinsonian drugs such as levodopa may alleviate some of the extrapyramidal features, but typically are less effective than in PD and more likely to be associated with adverse effects.

- Anticholinesterases are now the drugs of first choice for treating cognitive and neurobehavioural disturbance. In a placebo-controlled trial of rivastigmine, improvements were seen in hallucinations, delusions, apathy, indifference, anxiety and abberant motor behaviour, as well as in attention and other cognitive deficits.

Neuroleptics, including atypicals, are poorly tolerated and may cause severe and prolonged extrapyramidal reactions.

PARKINSON'S DISEASE AND DEMENTIA

Disturbances of cognition, insufficient to meet the criteria for dementia, are almost universal in PD. Patients typically have deficits in executive and spatial functions. However, these deficits do not always presage dementia.

The physical problems of PD, the treatments given for them and the frequently associated mood disturbance all make assessment difficult and dementia is often overlooked.

Epidemiology

- The point prevalence of dementia in people with PD is about 30% and the incidence is up to six times that in healthy people. The 8-year cumulative prevalence of PDD is nearly 80%. The relative contribution of concurrent AD, cortical Lewy Bodies, or other changes is much debated.

- Patients who become demented are usually older at onset of PD, have greater bradykinesia and gait disturbance, a more rapid downhill course and an unpredictable response to levodopa. Patients with tremor dominant PD are less likely to develop dementia.

Clinical features

- PDD may present as a cortical dementia resembling DLB, with fluctuating cognition and neuropsychiatric symptoms. Alternatively it present as a subcortical dementia, characterised by bradyphrenia and executive dysfunction.

- Nearly two thirds of PDD patients fulfil consensus criteria for probable DLB when the relative timing of presentation of symptoms is not taken into consideration.

Management

Treatment of the PD patient with dementia is especially difficult and choice and dose of drug therapy must be carefully balanced.

- Anti-Parkinsonian drugs tend to exacerbate confusion and may precipiate neuropsychiatric symptoms. Anticholinergic drugs should be stopped and dosage of other drugs reduced as much as possible. Neuroleptic drugs will worsen extrapyramidal signs and should be avoided.

- There is increasing evidence that anticholinesterase drugs may be of value in PDD, improving cognition, hallucinations, sleep disturbance and carer stress. In a few patients, Parkinsonism may be exacerbated.

- Presence of dementia is generally considered to be a contraindication to neurosurgical interventions.

FURTHER READING AND REFERENCES

Aarsland D, Ballard C, Larsen JP, et al. A comparative study of psychiatric symptoms in dementia with Lewy bodies and Parkinson's disease with and without dementia. Int J Geriatr Psychiatry 2001; 16: 528-36.

Ballard CG, O'Brien J, Lowery K, et al A prospective study of dementia with Lewy bodies. Age Ageing 1998; 27: 631-6.

Emre M. Dementia associated with Parkinson's disease. Lancet Neurol 2003; 2(4): 229-237.

Mahieux F, Fenelon G, Flahault A, et al. Neuropsychological prediction of dementia in Parkinson's disease. J Neurol Neurosurg Psychiatry 1999; 66: 297-304.

McKeith I, Galasko D, Kosaka K, et al. Consensus guidelines for the clinical and pathological diagnosis of dementia with Lewy bodies (DLB): report of the consortium on DLB international workshop. Neurology 1996; 47: 1113-1124.

McKeith IG, Perry EK, Perry RH. Report of the Second Dementia with Lewy body international workshop. Neurology 1999; 53: 902-5.

Rahkonen T, Eloniemi-Sulkava U, Rissanen S, et al. Dementia with Lewy bodies according to the consensus criteria in a general population aged 75 years or older. J Neurol Neurosurg Psychiatry 2003; 74: 720-4

Wilcock GK. Dementia with Lewy bodies. Lancet 2003; 362: 1689-90.

2.3

FRONTO-TEMPORAL DEMENTIA

Fronto-temporal dementia (FTD) is characterized by circumscribed atrophy of the frontal cortex and/or temporal cortex.

The clinical presentation is varied, but generally involves progressive personality and behavioural change and/or executive dysfunction and/or loss of language skills, with relatively preserved memory and visuospatial functions.

Background and terminology

- FTD is applied to various clinical syndromes, each of which reflects the topography of the pathological lesion within the brain, rather than any specific histopathological features. The term encompasses frontal lobe degeneration, frontal dementia, Pick's disease and primary progressive aphasia.

- Whilst several characteristic histological appearances arc described, associated with localized or symmetrical atrophy within the frontal and/or temporal lobes, none is associated with any particular clinical presentation. Definitive diagnosis therefore requires both a detailed clinical history and careful pathological examination.

- The acronym of "Pick's disease" is used by some to describe the clinical syndrome of frontal dementia, whereas others reserve its use for patients with the specific histopathological feature of ballooned neurones (Pick cells) and intracellular inclusion bodies (Pick bodies). Only a minority of FTD patients have typical Pick-type histopathology.

Epidemiology and genetics

- FTD is diagnosed in 2-3% of patients with dementia in unselected clinical series, but 5-15% in autopsy series. In younger people with dementia, FTD may account for up to 18% of cases.

- Presentation is usually before the age of 70 years and there may be a slight predominance of men. Mean survival time is about 6-9 years.

- About half of all cases have a family history. In familial cases, it tends to have a consistent presentation and course, though with great variation between families. Autosomal dominant transmission is usual and some cases have been linked to a missense mutation of the tau protein on chromosome 17 and others to a mutation on chromosome 3. The causes of sporadic FTD are so far unknown. The apolipoprotein e4 allele is not associated with FTD.

Neuropathology

- Pathological changes may be bilateral and symmetrical, affecting both frontal and temporal lobes (the posterior two-thirds of the superior temporal is characteristically better preserved than the rest of the temporal cortex)

- Sometimes the changes are more asymmetrical and localised, giving rise to a characteristic clinical picture (e.g. **primary progressive aphasia (PPA),** which reflects pathological change limited to the left perisylvian region).

- The amyloid plaques and neurofibrillary tangles characteristic of AD are rare or absent in FTD.

Histopathological subtypes of FTD include:

- **frontal lobe degeneration**, characterised by spongiform change and loss of large cortical nerve cells, with minimal gliosis and no inclusion bodies. These patients may have exactly the same clinical features and gross pathological appearance as in classical Pick's disease.

- **Pick's disease**, where there is no spongiform change, but widespread gliosis, marked astrocytosis and the characteristic Pick cells and Pick bodies (ballooned neurones with intracytoplasmic dense inclusion bodies) which stain positively for tau protein and ubiquitin.

- **FTD associated with spinal motor neurone disease**, with histology sharing features of both conditions.

Clinical features
Clinical presentation depends on the anatomic regions of the brain that are primarily affected, rather than the type of histopathology. Thus abnormalities reflect to a greater or lesser extent the functions of the frontal and/or temporal lobes.

- **Behavioural disturbance** is often the initial symptom, reflecting an orbitobasal frontal lobe focus of pathology. This may present as deterioration in social awareness and tact, disinhibition, coarsening of language, and neglect of personal hygeine and daily routine. The individual may become involved with the police because of some public misdemeanour, such as shoplifting or inappropriate sexual behaviour. There may be the development of compulsive collecting or repetitive or stereotyped rituals.

- **Personality and mood change.** There may be uncharacteristic and insensitive jokiness or rudeness and increasing selfishness and sometimes hypochondriasis. Patients may lose the ability to empathize with others and lack emotional warmth. Early loss of insight is characteristic.

Depression and anxiety may develop, but usually the overriding affect is one of apathy, lack of interest and remoteness.

- **Loss of frontal executive skills**, manifest as lack of initiative, poor insight, inattention and distractability. Typically there are problems with judgement, planning and abstraction and thinking becomes more rigid and inflexible.

- **Language dysfunction**. Generally speech is reduced in quantity, with word finding difficulty, lack of sponaneous conversation, concreteness and perseveration. Sometimes there may be a tendency to circumlocution, with many words, but little content. In **semantic dementia** there is a breakdown in the conceptual database that underlies language production and comprehension. There is usually progression through fluent aphasia to mutism. When progressive fluent or non-fluent speech disturbance presents in isolation and other cognitive and personality deficits do not develop for at least two years, the condition may be termed PPA.

- **Kluver-Bucy Syndrome** (hyperorality, visual agnosia and over response to visual stimuli) may develop.

- **Subtle neurological signs** may be present, especially release of 'primitive reflexes' such as snout, grasp and sucking reflexes. In the form of FTD associated with motor neurone disease, signs of pyramidal weakness, extensor plantar reflexes and muscle fasiculations (most easily seen over the deltoid muscle) accompany or follow the development of dementia. Rarely features of Parkinsonism may also occur.

Whatever the initial presentation of FTD, the onset is insidious and then slowly progresses. Memory and visuospatial functions are relatively preserved until late in the disease and patients usually look and are physically well. Urinary incontinence may be an early feature, but other self-care abilities tend to be maintained and patients with well established FTD may still be generally independent. Eating disturbances, such as a tendency to overindulge, or a change in food preferences typically with an especial liking for sweets, may lead to significant weight change.

Assessment and diagnosis

- Diagnosis will be suggested by the history of behavioural change and/or progressive language disturbance. Marked problems in some areas contrast with preserved ability in others. Reliable information must be sought from family and friends, as the history from the patient is often highly unreliable.

- Scores on simple screening tests such as MMSE may be misleading, as orientation, memory and visuo-constructional skills are likely to be relatively intact until late in the disease. Specific tests of language and/or frontal executive function skill will be impaired. There are often difficultities with attention and simple problem solving, a tendency to concrete rather than abstract thinking and to perseverate on testing, with problems shifting from one task to the next. Physical examination is unremarkable except for the presence of primitive reflexes.

- CT (or MRI) scanning typically will show localised cortical atrophy of the frontal and/or temporal lobes, with enlargement of the frontal and /or temporal horns of the lateral ventricles. This is asymmetrical in about 50% of patients and then usually more conspicuous on the left than right side. Scans may be normal early in the disease.

- SPECT (or PET) scanning is useful when atrophy is inconspicuous and to complement structural imaging. Characteristically this will demonstrate anterior frontal and/or temporal hypoperfusion, which may be unilateral or bilateral.

- The EEG is usually normal throughout the course of the illness.

Many disorders can disrupt frontal lobe function and ultimately the diagnosis of Pick's disease and frontal lobe dementia can be confirmed only at autopsy.

Table *Causes of frontal lobe syndromes*

Primary frontal degenerative disorders

- *Pick's disease*
- *Frontal lobe degeneration*
- *Frontotemporal dementia with motor neurone disease*
- *Progressive subcortical gliosis*
- *Familial FTD disorders*

Other degenerative disorders

- *Alzheimer's disease*
- *Corticobasal degeneration*
- *Parkinson's disease*
- *Progressive supranuclear palsy*
- *Huntington's disease*

Vascular disease

- *Frontal lobe infarct or aneurysm*
- *Lacunar state*
- *Binswanger's disease*
- *CADASIL*

Other conditions

- *Multiple sclerosis*
- *Tumour*
- *Head injury*
- *Hydrocephalus*
- *HIV*
- *Prion disease*
- *Syphilis*

Management

- Selective serotonin reuptake inhibitors, such as paroxetine, may help anxiety and repetitive, ritualistic behaviours. Valproic acid and atypical neuroleptics, such as quetiapine may help to calm agitated patients. However, there is some evidence that patients with FTD may, as in DLB, be particularly sensitive to the extrapyramidal side effects of neuroleptics and they should be used cautiously, starting at low doses and avoiding depot prepartions.

- Depression and apathy tend to be resistant to treatment. Anticholinesterases have not proved useful and there are anecdotal reports that they may increase agitation.

- The marked personality and behavioural changes early in the course of the illness often create major difficulties in caring for patients at home and need for institutional care occurs earlier than in most other dementias. Patients tend to adopt their own rigid routine and it is up to others to adapt to accommodate it.

FURTHER READING AND REFERENCES

Binetti G, Growdon JH, Vonsattel J-PG. Pick's disease. In Growdon JH, Rossor MN (eds.) The dementias. London, Butterworth-Heinemann 1998..

Levy ML, Miller BL, Cummings JL. Frontal and frontotemporal dementia. . In Growdon JH, Rossor MN (eds.) The dementias. London, Butterworth-Heinemann 1998.

Lund and Manchester Groups. Clinical and neuropathological criteria for frontotemporal dementia. J Neurology Neurosurg Psychiatry 1994; 57: 416-8.

Neary D, Snowden JS, Gustafson L, et al. Frontotemporal lobar degeneration: a consensus on clinical diagnostic criteria. Neurology 1998; 51: 1546-1554

Snowden JS, Bathgate D, Varma A, et al. Distinct behavioural profiles in frontotemporal dementia and semantic dementia. J Neurol Neurosurg Psychiatry 2001; 70: 323-332.

2.4

OTHER DEGENERATIVE BRAIN DISEASE

PROGRESSIVE SUPRANUCLEAR PALSY

A variety of Parkinson's plus syndromes have been described in recent years and many are associated with symptoms of dementia. Progressive supranuclear palsy (PSP), or Steele Richardson Osliewski syndrome, is the best defined. It is an uncommon condition, usually presenting in the 50s or 60s.

Pathology

The pathological changes of atrophy, neuronal loss and gliosis are found in the subcortical and mid brain regions, with sparing of the cerebral cortex. The degenerating neurones contain neurofibrillary tangles, but these are not twisted as is characteristic of Alzheimer's disease and there are no senile plaques.

Clinical features

There is a variable age of onset and the initial symptoms are often mistaken for Parkinson's disease. As the condition develops, the diagnostic features become apparent:

- **rigidity** of neck and upper trunk, giving a mask-like, staring, 'surprised' expression to the face with loss of blinking. There is a strikingly erect posture and the rigidity is symmetrical. Whilst gait disturbance and instability develop early, arm swing tends to be preserved until late in the disease.

- **supranuclear opthalmoplegia** (progressive paralysis of vertical eye movements, especially downward gaze) occurs early. This leads to unsteadiness and falls, difficulty reading, eating and general clumsiness.

- **pseudobulbar palsy**, leading to dysarthria and problems with swallowing.

- **slowly progressive, subcortical dementia**. This probably arises from damage to inter-connected subcortical and frontal lobe structures, leading to reduced arousal and motivation. The characteristic features are forgetfulness, personality change (particularly apathy and depression), poor calculation and abstraction skills and marked slowing of cognitive processes. Often, if allowed sufficient time, patients will eventually respond to questions correctly. Language and visuo-spatial ability is generally unimpaired. The concept of subcortical dementia was first based on evaluation of people with PSP.

NINDS diagnostic criteria require onset over age 40, a progressive course, bradykinesia and supranuclear palsy, together with three of either dysarthria, dysphagia, extended neck posture, minimal or no tremor, pyramidal tract signs, early gait disturbance, frequent falls and more axial than limb rigidity. Cerebellar signs, polyneuropathy and autonomic dysfunction should be absent.

The established disease contrasts sharply with both the typically cortical dementia of AD and the stooped, tremulous posture of idiopathic PD.

Diagnosis and treatment.

This is essentially based on clinical skills. Neuroimaging is usually normal, though SPECT scanning may show an anterior perfusion defect. Response to dopaminergic drugs is disappointing and anticholinesterase drugs are ineffective.

CORTICOBASAL DEGENERATION

This is an uncommon form of dementia of unknown cause that presents with cognitive impairment and aymmetrical motor symptoms. Age of onset is usually greater than 60, with no sex difference, familial tendency or geographic clustering.

Pathology

There is asymmetrical frontoparietal atrophy and gliosis. Microscopically there are cortical ballooned neurones with resistance to staining (neuronal achromosia) and degeneration of the substantia nigra and subcortical nuclei.

Clinical features

There is a wide variety of presentations, with some patients first exhibiting motor symptoms and others presenting with cognitive impairment. Misdiagnosis is very common.

- Motor symptoms are nearly always aymmetrical and often present as a stiff hand or arm, with problems writing and carrying out activities requiring fine movement. The rigidity, bradykinesia and postural instability may suggest PD. Rest tremor is usually absent. The 'alien limb' is characteristic and may progress to a flexed, dystonic posturing of the distal joints. Myoclonus is often present.

- Cognition appears intact early in the illness, but there is then progressive dementia, often with prominent dysphasia.

Management

This is mainly palliative. Response to dopaminergic drugs is slight. Clonazepam may help rigidity and myoclonus. The condition progresses over 5-y years to a state of profound rigidity.

Table *Key features in differential diagnosis of dementias associated with motor signs*

	Motor features	**Cognitive features**
Parkinson's disease	Rest tremor, asymmetry, good response to levodopa	Dementia develops several years after motor signs
Dementia with Lewy bodies	Parkinsonism usually mild early in disease; symmetrical; rest tremor absent	Dementia develops concurrently or before motor signs; marked fluctuations; visual hallucinations
Progressive supranuclear palsy	Supranuclear gaze palsy; axial rigidity; falls	Frontal executive dysfunction; typical subcortical dementia
Cortico-basal degeneration	Asymmetriy; alien hand; myoclonus	Cognitive loss follows motor loss; aphasia
Normal pressure hydrocephalus	Gait apraxia; incontinence	Marked memory deficit; cortical deficits uncommon
Motor neurone disease	Upper and lower motor neurone signs	Frontal dementia (precedes motor signs)
Huntington's disease	Involuntary movements; gait disturbance	Frontal executive dysfunction, language preserved
Binswanger's disease	Marche a petits pas, pyramidal tract signs, lower body Parkinsonism	Patchy cognitive impairment; marked psychomotor slowing

HUNTINGTON'S DISEASE

This is a progressive familial condition mainly affecting the basal ganglia. It is an autosomal dominant disorder with complete penetrance, the mutant gene having been identified on the long arm of chromosome 4. As it is genetically transmitted, cases tend to cluster with an overall prevalence of about 50 per million. Prevalence is highest in those of Western European origin.

Pathology

There is selective atrophy of the caudate nucleus, globus pallidus and putamen. Microscopy shows severe loss of small neurons and gliosis, which correlates with severity of dementia. These neurons particularly contain the neurotransmitter gamma aminobutyric acid (GABA). There is also cell loss in the frontal cortex and sometimes more generalised neuronal loss and cortical atrophy.

Clinical features

Symptoms usually develop in middle age, but can present as late as 60 or 70 years. There is a triad of clinical features:

- Initial symptoms of fidgetiness and clumsiness progress to chorea and other involuntary movements. There is prominent gait disturbance. Motor involvement also causes progressive dysarthria and dysphagia

- Depression (and suicide) and alterations in behaviour, typically with delusions, disinhibition and personality change, are common.

- There is a typically subcortical dementia. Reasoning, judgement and problem-solving abilities most noticeably decline, together with a progressive failure of memory and visuospatial ability. Communication becomes increasingly difficult as motor symptoms become more advanced, but language is relatively preserved.

The condition tends to have a remarkably stereotyped natural history within an individual family and in families with late age of onset, dementia is often less severe. Death occurs between 10 to 20 years after onset of symptoms.

Diagnosis and management

Although the diagnosis is usually made clinically, this can be confirmed by genetic testing. This also allows for presymptomatic (and prenatal) testing, with the attendant legal, ethical and psychosocial challenges.

PRION DEMENTIA (CREUTZFELDT-JAKOB DISEASE, GERSTMANN-STRAUSSLER SYNDROME)

These rare, usually rapidly progressive dementing illnesses, affect both sexes with onset usually after age 55. The incidence is about 1 per 2 million population per year, with occasional clusters. New variant CJD is so far mainly restricted to the UK and has a younger onset and slightly slower course (median survival of 2 years versus 1 year for classical CJD).

Pathology

The prion diseases arise from abnormal folding of a normal brain protein into a pathological isoform. In humans, prion disease may be:

- Familial (associated with autosomal dominant prion protein gene mutations, resulting in characteristic phenotypes including Gerstmann-Straussler syndrome and fatal familial insomnia)

- Sporadic (from spontaneous production of pathogenic prion protein, resulting in classical CJD)

- Iatrogenic (including transmission of pathogenic prion protein in pooled human pituitary-derived growth hormone, corneal grafts and neurosurgical and electrophysiological instruments)

- Transmissable (classically as Kuru, due to cannibalsim and recently as new variant CJD, transmitted in beef infected with bovine spongiform encephalopathy)

Microscopically, the principal features are spongiform change of cerebral grey matter, neuronal loss and astrocytic hypertrophy. These are accompanied by the presence of protease-resistant, amyloid-like (prion protein) plaques, particularly in the cerebellum. Pathological disease-associated prion protein can be identified not only in the central nervous system, but also in olfactory-nerve tissue and in some patients in spleen and skeletal-muscle. Extraneural prion protein appears to correlate with a longer duration of disease.

Clinical features

Subacute (85%) chronic (10%) and amyotrophic (5%) presentations are described.

- Initial symptoms and signs are variable, but fatigue, forgetfulness, speech disturbance and motor abnormalities are common, with rapid progressive cognitive impairment. Pyramidal, extrapyramidal and cerebellar features may accompany dementia. Within a few months this may lead to myoclonus, fits and eventually a state of akinetic mutism.

- New variant CJD presents with behavioural change and progressive ataxia, accompanying cognitive decline.

- The rapidity of developing dementia in prion disease is characteristic. An EEG typically shows generalised repetitive triphasic complexes with suppression of background rhythms, but this finding may be transient and its absence does not exclude diagnosis. CT scan is usually normal. A tonsillar biopsy may demonstrate prion protein in variant CJD.

Management

There is no effective medical treatment. Precautions are needed when handling pathological material to prevent accidental transmission of the disease.

OTHER CONDITIONS

Motor neurone disease may rarely be associated with a severe and rapidly progressive frontal-type dementia. Normally, however, cognitive function is not affected and it is the progressive physical problems that lead to severe dependency.

Multiple sclerosis is often associated with mild and very slowly progressive cognitive impairment, but sometimes the condition can lead to dementia, usually subcortical in nature. Interpretation of cognitive tests is complicated by the presence of motor and sensory deficits, poor vision, emotional disturbance and a tendency to tire easily. Patients with the chronic progressive form of the illness show more deterioration in cognitive ability than those with the remitting-relapsing form (as cognition is static between relapses).

Progressive subcortical gliosis presents as a very slowly progressive dementia, usually misdiagnosed in life as AD or PSP. Pathologically there is diffuse cerebral atrophy and astrocytosis throughout the cortex.

FURTHER READING AND REFERENCES

Albert ML, Feldman RG, Willis AL. The subcortical dementia of progressive supranuclear palsy. J Neurol Neurosurg Psychiatry 1974: 37; 121-130.

Collinge J. Human prion diseases and bovine spongiform encephalopathy (BSE). Hum Mol Genet 1997; 6: 1699-705.

Folstein SE, Leigh RJ, Parhad IM, et al. The diagnosis of Huntington's disease. Neurology 1986; 36: 421-30.

Hauw J, Daniel SE, Dickson D, et al. Preliminary NINDS neuropathologic criteria for Steele Richardson Olszewski syndrome (progressive supranuclear palsy). Neurology 1994; 44: 2015-9.
Jones AL, Wood JD, Harper PS. Huntington disease: advances in molecular and cell biology. J Inherited Metabolic Dis 1997; 20: 125-38.
Martin JB and Gusella JF. Huntington's disease: pathogenesis and management. New Eng J Med 1986; 315: 1267-76.
Schneider JA, Watts RL, Gearing M, et al. Corticobasal degeneration: neuropathologic and clinical heterogeneity. Neurology 1997; 48: 959-69.
Sagar HJ. Parkinsonian syndromes associated with dementia. In: Growden JH, Rossor MN (eds) The dementias. London, Butterworth-Heinemann 1998.
Wexler N. Huntington's disease. Curr Opin Neurology Neurosurg. 1998; 1: 319-23.
Will R and Zeidler M. Diagnosing Creutzfeldt-Jakob disease. BMJ 1996; 313: 833-834.

2.5

VASCULAR DEMENTIA

The term 'vascular dementia' encompasses dementia arising from any disturbance of blood supply to the brain and is preferable to 'multi-infarct dementia' that is considered to be too restrictive. Even the validity of the diagnosis of VaD is challenged and alternatives such as 'vascular cognitive impairment' have been proposed.

Epidemiology

- In the Western World, VaD generally is believed to be the second most common cause of dementia (after AD), but worldwide it may be the most common cause. VaD is a relatively more important cause of dementia in men than in women and in people of Afro Caribbean and East Asian origin.

- Studies of prevalence of VaD in clinical and pathological series vary widely in their estimates. The prevalence of pure VaD is likely to be low (perhaps 10-20%), but the overall contribution of vascular disease to cognitive decline and dementia may be very significant (perhaps relevant in the majority of cases). It is likely that vascular disease and degenerative disease often interact with one lowering the threshold for another (so called 'mixed dementia').

- Prevalence and incidence rise exponentially with age, at least until age 90 years, though the rise is less steep than for AD.

Classification

The main sub-types of vascular dementia are:

- **multiple cortical infarction (cortical vascular dementia)**, generally associated with large artery, atheromatous or thromboembolic disease.

- **strategic infarct dementia**, arising from small, critically located lesions, for example in the thalamus (particularly if bilateral), head of the caudate nucleus, medial temporal lobe (commonly the hippocampus), or angular gyrus.

- **the lacunar state**, with multiple subcortical lacunes **(small vessel dementia or subcortical vascular dementia)**. These small, deep cerebral infarcts occur particularly in the basal ganglia, thalamus, brainstem and internal capsule and are secondary to occlusion of end arteriolar vessels, which have no collateral anastomoses. Binswanger's disease, often associated with uncontrolled hypertension leads to ischaemic demyelination in the periventricular arterial end zones, with both complete and incomplete microinfarction.

- **haemodynamic dementia**, secondary to hypoperfusion associated with cardiac arrest, systemic haemorrhage, or surgery.

Other less common causes of vascular dementia include:

- **haemorrhagic dementia**

- **cerebral vasculitis** (either as a primary disorder or associated with collagen disorders, malignancy or drugs)

- **hereditary agiopathies** (e.g. familial amyloid angiopathy and cerebral autosomal dominant arteriopathy with subcortical infarcts and leukoencephalopathy, CADASIL)

- **mitochondrial disease** (mitochondrial encephalopathy, lactic acidosis and stroke-like episodes, MELAS).

Aetiology

Some degree of cerebral atheroma is almost ubiquitous in later life, but this does not always lead to symptoms. Similarly many strokes do not significantly affect higher mental function. Nevertheless, a stroke increases risk of developing dementia about none-fold compared to non-stroke patients. The prognosis for people with stroke and co-existent dementia is much worse than for those with normal cognitive function.

Factors which appear to be of importance in deciding if cerebrovascular disease will cause dementia appear to be:

- the total volume of brain tissue which is infarcted. The number of lesions is less important. Extensive white matter lesions appear to make dementia more likely.

- the bilaterality of lesions (perhaps because memory is bilaterally represented)

- the strategic location of the lesions. Often implicated are infarctions in the hippocampus and adjacent limbic structures, or in the corpus callosum and deep frontal white matter.

The risk factors for developing vascular dementia are assumed to be similar to those for stroke, namely age, hypertension, diabetes and previous stroke or myocardial infarction. Typically patients who have an underlying predisposition to vascular disease will be more likely to have a vascular contribution to their dementia.

Clinical features

- Diagnosis is not always easy and the condition is probably regularly over- and under-diagnosed. Even when vascular disease is demonstrated clinically and radiologically, it will be uncertain if the observed vascular change is the cause of dementia, a contributory factor, or purely coincidental.

- Typically the onset of vascular dementia is abrupt, with a patchy distribution of cognitive deficits and subsequent stepwise downward progression. When there is an obvious time relationship between clinical evidence of an infarct and development of dementia, it is more apparent that the two are likely to be related. However, many infarcts are too small to produce a distinct clinical incident and it is their summation that leads to cognitive impairment. The dementia will then have an insidious onset and gradual course similar to Alzheimer's disease.

- Focal neurological signs and symptoms, especially asymmetrical limb weakness or deep tendon reflexes, an extensor plantar response, visual field defects and gait disturbance are suggestive of a vascular cause for dementia.

- Relative preservation of insight, changes in mood and emotional lability and early urinary incontinence are characteristic.

- The lacunar state is typically associated with pyramidal and extrapyramidal signs and pseudobulbar palsy, leading to dysarthria and dysphagia. There is often a stiff, small stepping gait (marche a petits pas).

- Subcortical dementia, due to ischaemic involvement of deep white matter, presents with bradyphrenia, apathy and poor concentration and problem solving abilities. There is typically a specific difficulty in memory retrieval. The condition may suggest Parkinsonism.

Diagnosis

- Diagnosis of VaD will be suggested by the history and clinical presentation, often supported by results of neuroimaging.

- The Hachinski Ischaemia Score uses a variety of clinical parameters to differentiate between multi infarct dementia and Alzheimer's disease. A low score (4 or less) makes a vascular aetiology unlikely. The higher the score, the greater the likelihood of stroke disease. Despite widespread reservations about the reliability and validity of the Ischaemia Score and numerous modifications, it remains clinically useful.

- Neuroimaging is helpful in providing evidence of vascular disease, but cannot be diagnostic on its own. Cortical and subcortical infarction is usually clearly visible on magnetic resonance imaging (MRI) and to a lesser degree with computed tomography (CT). White matter changes or leukoaraiosis (areas of high signal intensity in the white matter on MRI or decreased density on CT images) are often seen symmetrically distributed adjacent to the ventricles or deep in the white matter. However, they are of uncertain significance, being found in many healthy elderly subjects and a third or more of Alzheimer's patients. It is suggested that more than 25% involvement of the white matter supports a vascular aetiology for dementia.

- Operational criteria to define vascular dementia have been proposed by several groups including the NINDS-AIREN Workshop. In recognition that some vascular events are clinically silent, CT or MRI scans showing ischaemic lesions are a necessary part of most definitions, but it is also recognised that there are no features on brain imaging that make the diagnosis of vascular dementia certain.

Management

- Medical intervention should concentrate on treating risk factors for vascular disease (e.g. hypertension, diabetes mellitus, smoking, hypercholesterolaemia and cardiac disease) in order to prevent further cerebral damage.

- Use of prophylactic low dose aspirin or other antiplatelet drug is likely to reduce risk of further vascular events and therefore slow symptom progression. Oral anticoagulation should be considered in those with a clear source of emboli, such as valvular heart disease or atrial fibrillation. Age should not influence the decision to start warfarin, but risk of falls and problems with ensuring compliance may make anticoagulation unsafe.

- Corticosteroids or immunosuppressant treatment may be indicated in those with active inflammatory arterial disease and may be dramatically effective.

- Carotid artery surgery should be considered in those with greater than 70% stenosis and relatively mild cognitive deficits.

- Anticholinesterase drugs may have benefits comparable to those seen in pure AD, with improvement in cognition and maintenance of activities of daily living and global function. There is also some clinical trial evidence to support efficacy of memantine in VaD. The usefulness of other medication, including nimodipine and gingko biloba is questionable.

FURTHER READING AND REFERENCES

Carlson LA, Gottfries CG, Winblad B (eds.). Vascular Dementia. Dementia 1994: 5: 129-214.

O'Brien JO, Ames D, Gustafson L, Chiu E, Folstein MF. Cerebrovascular Disease, Cognitive Impairment and Dementia, 2nd edition. London, Martin Dunitz 2003.

Erkinjuntti T, Gauthier S. Vascular Cognitive Impaiment. London, Martin Dunitz 2002

Hachinski VC, et al. Multi-infarct dementia; a cause of mental deterioration in the elderly. Lancet 1974; ii: 207-210.

Roman G, et al. Vascular dementia: diagnostic criteria for research studies. Report of the NINDS-AIREN International Workshop. Neurology 1993; 43: 250-260.

Roman G. Vascular dementia revisited; pathogenesis, treatment and prevention. Med Clin North America 2002; 86: 477-499.

Stewart R. Vascular dementia: a diagnosis running out of time. Br J Psychiatry 2002; 180: 152-156.

Zekry D, Hauw JJ, Gold G. Mixed dementia: epidemiology, diagnosis and treatment. JAGS 2002; 50: 1431-8.

2.6

OTHER CAUSES OF DEMENTIA

NORMAL PRESSURE HYDROCEPHALUS

Normal pressure hydrocephalus (NPH) is characterised by ventricular enlargement, with normal or only intermittently raised cerebrospinal fluid pressure. Often the condition develops secondary to previous brain pathology, such as meningitis, head injury, neurosurgery, or subarachnoid haemorrhage. In these circumstances it is assumed that meningeal fibrosis interrupts CSF drainage from the subarachnoid space. In up to half of cases, NPH has an uncertain origin, though vascular mechanisms are thought to be important. Symptoms are attributed to the stretching of nerve fibres around the dilated ventricles.

Clinical features

NPH is most often seen in people in their 60s or 70s. Classically it presents with a triad of symptoms of insidious onset and progressing over a few months:

- **dementia** (particularly fluctuating memory disturbance, mental slowing, dyscalculia, apathy, loss of insight, confabulation and emotional blunting). Behavioural disturbance is uncommon
- **gait disturbance**, ranging from mild, symmetrical clumsiness, to unsteady shuffling, to gross apraxia. This may lead to frequent falls and especial difficulty in initiating, turning and climbing stairs. It may precede other symptoms and signs.

- **urinary incontinence**, usually the last symptom to develop and characteristically of little concern to the patient.

- Other common features include fatigue, weakness, dizziness and fits.

Diagnosis.

- NPH may be suspected when CT scan shows ventricular dilatation that is disproportionate to the degree of atrophy. A midline tumour must be excluded.

- CSF pressure on lumbar puncture is normal, but continuous monitoring of intracranial pressure shows it to be intermittently raised ('B waves').

- A positive response (e.g. fewer steps to walk 18 metres, improved reaction time) to removal of CSF (30-40 ml) by repeated lumbar puncture (at 2-3 day intervals) is sometimes used to predict those patients most likely to respond to surgical intervention. There is only limited evidence that this is reliable.

- Radionucleide cisternography (RISA scan) may show penetration of isotope into the ventricles, with reduced collection in the superior sagittal sinus, but this finding is not specific to NPH and poorly predicts response to surgery.

Management

Surgical intervention may help symptoms and stop progression by inserting a ventricular-caval/peritoneal shunt with a one-way low-pressure valve to divert CSF. Unfortunately, response is unpredictable, with benefit being seen in 30-50% of patients. Reduction of ventricular size after shunting is not predictive of clinical improvement. Complications (blocked shunts, infection, subdural haematoma, seizures) are common. The mortality rate associated with surgery may be up to 25%.

Patients with acute onset of symptoms and predominant gait disturbance and those with secondary hydrocephalus seem to have the best outcome after shunting. Those with severe dementia and evidence of atrophy on CT scan have a poor outcome. If successful, dementia and incontinence rapidly improve, but gait disturbance recovers more slowly.

If untreated, NPH may slowly progress to a state of total immobility and mutism.

ALCOHOL-RELATED DEMENTIA

Up to half of middle aged and older chronic alcohol abusers have some cognitive impairment and about 10% become demented. This may arise because of:

- direct neurotoxic effects of alcohol or its metabolites, causing alcoholic dementia
- indirectly by poor nutrition associated with alcoholism leading to vitamin deficiency. In particular, thiamine deficiency causes Wernicke-Korsakoff's syndrome.

Lesser degrees of cognitive impairment are very common, as is evidence of ventricular enlargement and cerebral and cerebellar atrophy on CT Scan. Compared to abstainers, even moderate social drinkers are more likely to show subtle cognitive deficits of abstract and adaptive reasoning and other executive skills. Just as individuals vary in their susceptibility to acute effects of alcohol, so do they to its chronic effects.

The elderly brain appears especially vulnerable to the effects of alcohol. This is presumably because of pre-existing neuronal loss and lowered functional reserve. Indeed, it is sometimes suggested that the effects of chronic alcohol ingestion parallel the effects of normal ageing.

Other factors predisposing to the development of alcohol-associated cognitive impairment include lower premorbid intellect, recurrent head trauma, liver disease and poor nutritional status. Risk is also closely correlated with estimated lifetime alcohol consumption (duration and average intake) and pattern of drinking (steady versus binge). A family history is often present.

Alcoholic dementia accounts for 1-2% of all dementia. It presents with diffuse cognitive impairment, similar to degenerative dementia. The DSM-IV criteria refer to alcohol-induced persisting dementia, characterised by dementia with evidence from history, examination or investigations that deficits are aetiologically related to the persisting effects of alcohol. A careful history should distinguish the chronic alcoholic who has developed cognitive impairment and fulfils criteria for dementia, from the person whose dementia due to some other cause has resulted in uncontrolled alcohol intake.

Characteristics of alcoholic dementia include:

- There tend to be prominent deficits in executive tasks (e.g. abstraction, problem solving), recall and recognition, and visuo-spatial tasks. Verbal skills often are relatively preserved. Labile mood, hallucinations and delusions are common features.

- Physical examination may show evidence of liver disease and alcohol abuse.

- Cerebral atrophy particularly involves the frontal lobes and can be demonstrated on neuroimaging. There may be evidence of old head injury or subdural haematoma.

- Alcoholic dementia progresses with continued drinking, but may partially reverse if abstinence from alcohol can be attained. Frontal lobe dysfunction means that this is seldom easy. Any recovery may take months or years and is not as rapid or significant in older alcoholics as it is in younger abusers. Involving family and friends may help to maintain abstinence and ensure a good diet and facilitate return to day-to-day life.

Wernicke-Korsakoff's syndrome arises secondary to thiamine deficiency and is most often associated with alcoholism.

- It classically presents with encephalopathy, predominantly anterograde amnesia and confabulation, opthalmoplegia and cerebellar ataxia. Not all features are always present.

- Pathologically there is periventricular and periaqueductal cell loss with micro haemorrhages. Atrophy of the mammillary bodies and dorsomedial nucleus of the thalamus can be seen on MRI Scan.

- If there is any suspicion of alcohol abuse, patients should be given thiamine, which will arrest and may partly reverse the symptoms. Only a fifth of patients fully recover and over half are left with permanent Korsakoff's psychosis, characterised by poor new learning ability, confabulation, apathy and loss of insight.

SUBDURAL HAEMATOMA

Subdural haematoma usually follows head injury, though this is not always severe or even recalled. It is more frequently identified in chronic alcoholics. Sometimes a subdural haematoma may develop spontaneously in patients on anticoagulants or with bleeding disorders. Many are unrecognised in life.

- Characteristically subdural haematomas lead to a fluctuating level of consciousness and mental impairment that varies from day to day. A chronic subdural haematoma can cause more consistent and severe dementia, but it is an uncommon cause of progressive intellectual loss. Signs of raised intracranial pressure may be present.

- Whilst in the early stage, a haematoma is clearly visible on CT Scan, it becomes isodense with the surrounding brain after 14 days and may require contrast enhancement before it can be seen.

- Surgical evacuation is potentially curative, but outcome is often poor, especially when the condition is long-standing.

DEMENTIA PUGILISTICA

Boxing often results in long term brain damage, which may not become apparent until 30 or 40 years after the end of the boxer's career. Number of fights and length of career seem to be more important than number of knock-outs. The risk of developing brain injury may be as high as 80-90%.

- Poor memory, slowness of thought, difficulty in speech and unsteadiness are the most common symptoms. Dysarthria and cerebellar, pyramidal and extrapyramidal features tend to occur early, followed by progressive cognitive impairment.

- Pathological features include generalised cortical atrophy and cavum septum pallucidum (also visible on CT scan), together with loss of pigment in the substantia nigra and neurofibrillary tangles in the neocortex. Senile plaques and Lewy bodies are absent.

- Treatment is palliative.

BRAIN TUMOURS

The incidence of brain tumours rises with age. In elderly patients they are often metastatic and supratentorial and the commonest primary pathologies are meningiomas and malignant glial tumours.

- Slow growing tumours, especially in the frontal lobe and corpus callosum, may present with gradual cognitive impairment and retardation, without lateralising neurological signs. They can then easily be confused with presentation of a primary dementia. Focal cortical deficits, such as dysphasia or dyspraxia arising from a lesion in the temporal or parietal lobes can also trap the unwary.

- Some systemic malignancies can also cause neurobehavioural symptoms, even in the absence of metastatic deposits. Ectopic hormone production, progressive multifocal leucoencephalopathy and the immune-based paraneoplastic syndrome, most commonly related to small cell carcinoma of the lung, may all be implicated.

- Treatment depends on the underlying pathology. Surgical resection of symptomatic meningiomas can be particularly successful. Neurosurgery and whole-brain irradiation can themselves sometimes result in a dementia syndrome.

NEUROSYPHILITIC DEMENTIA

Neurosyphilis was once a very common cause of dementia, but is now rare. The latent period between infection and presentation is up to 40 years.

- Clinical presentation nowadays is often modified by inadequate chance treatment with antibiotics. Depression or loss of inhibitions and inappropriate social behaviour tend to be early features, progressing to generalised severe intellectual impairment. Focal neurological signs, including Argyll Robertson pupils, are usual.

- Symptoms will respond to an appropriate course of penicillin, though cognitive impairment does not improve as rapidly as other neurological manifestations.

AIDS-ASSOCIATED DEMENTIA

Dementia may develop as a late complication of Acquired Immunodeficiency Syndrome (AIDS), either as a feature of human immunodeficiency virus (HIV) encephalopathy, or through opportunistic infection or lymphoma affecting the central nervous system.

Over half of AIDS patients have some cognitive impairment prior to their death and at post mortem, 80% have pathological markers of HIV infection in the brain. However, prominent dementia affects only 15-20%. Risk is greatest in those with a low haemoglobin, older age at onset and in those with a CD4 count below 100. With recent therapeutic advances, HIV/AIDS dementia may be becoming less prevalent.

- Clinically, motor symptoms and focal neurological signs often accompany the dementia, which may be apparent before other signs of AIDS. Subcortical dementia, with mental slowing and impaired frontal function, is most characteristic of AIDS-associated dementia and also of toxoplamosis infection. Deficits on tests of planning, motor speed and nonverbal memory are often seen. A more mixed picture of language disturbance and executive dysfunction is seen with brain cryptococcosis. There may be prominent neuropsychiatric symptoms of apathy, social withdrawal and personality change. Symptoms may progress to akinetic mutism.

- Pathologically, HIV encephalopathy is associated with generalised cerebral atrophy and a diffuse loss of myelin in the deep white matter. The mechanism of neuronal damage involves expression of destructive viral proteins on the surface of macrophages in the brain and production of neurotoxic cytokines

- HIV serology is positive and toxoplasmosis, mycobacterial, cryptococcal and syphilitic infection must be excluded. There will usually be evidence of severe immunosuppression. Neuroimaging may show cerebral atrophy and white matter lesions, or evidence of CNS infection.

- Without treatment, AIDS dementia progresses rapidly and typical survival is only a few months. Retroviral therapy slows cognitive decline.

METABOLIC DEMENTIA

Many metabolic and hormonal disturbances may lead to disturbed consciousness and behavioural impairment. Most commonly this is a subacute delirious state, rather than a true dementia.

Traditionally **thyroid disease, pernicious anaemia, hypoglycaemia, hyperparathyroidism, hypopituitarism, cerebral anoxia, possibly folic acid deficiency and renal and hepatic failure** have been listed as causes of 'reversible dementia.'

Prompt treatment of metabolic disturbance is nearly always appropriate. Whilst it may not reverse all existing deficits, it will certainly modify further deterioration.

Other very rare metabolic causes of dementia include:

- **Wilson's disease**. This is an autosomal recessive inherited disorder of copper metabolism, characterised by low serum copper and caeruloplasmin, with elevated urinary copper excretion. Kayser-Fleischer rings in the cornea are demonstrated by slit lamp examination. Cognitive symptoms are accompanied by motor signs.

- **Storage diseases (e.g. Niemann-Pick disease type C, Kufs disease)** may present from infancy to early middle age. Dementia accompanies a wide variety of neurological signs. Diagnosis is made on biopsy of skin, bone marrow or liver.

- **Metachromatic leukodystrophy**. An autosomal recessive disorder of myelin metabolism caused by lack of the enzyme arylsulphatase A. A frontal lobe syndrome typically accompanies motor symptoms, emotional lability and peripheral neuropathy.

FURTHER READING AND REFERENCES

Adhiyaman V, Asghar M, Ganeshram KN, et al. Chronic subdural haematoma in the elderly. Postgrad Med J. 2002;78(916):71-5.

Editorial. Normal-pressure hydrocephalus. Lancet 1990 : i ; 22.

Erlanger DM, Kutner KC, Barth JT, et al. Neuropsychology of sports-related head injury: Dementia Pugilistica to Post Concussion Syndrome. Clin Neuropsychol1999;13:193-209

Esmonde T, Cooke S. Shunting for normal pressure hydrocephalus. Cochrane Database Syst Rev. 2002; (3): CD003157.

Graff-Radford NR, Godersky JC, Jones MP. Variables predicting surgical outcome in symptomatic hydrocephalus in the elderly. Neurology 1989; 39: 1601-4.

Grant I. Alcohol and the brain: neuropsychological correlates. J Consulting Clin Psychol 1987; 55: 310-324.

Hebb AO, Cusimano MD. Idiopathic normal pressure hydrocephalus: a systematic review of diagnosis and outcome. Neurosurgery. 2001; 49: 1166-84

Jordan BD. Chronic traumatic brain injury associated with boxing. Semin Neurol. 2000;20: 179-85.

King MB. Alcohol abuse and dementia. Int J Geriatr Psychiatry 1986:1; 31-36.

Lipton SA. Neuropathegenesis of acquired immunodeficiency syndrome dementia. Curr Opin Neurol 1997; 10: 247-53.

Price RW. Neurological complications of HIV infection. Lancet 1996; 348: 445-52.

Smith DM, Atkinson RM. Alcoholism and dementia. Int J Addict 1995; 30 (suppl 13-14): 1843-69.

Vanneste J, Augustin PA, Dirven C, et al. Shunting normal pressure hydrocephalus: do the benefits outweigh the risks? Neurology 1992; 42: 54-9.

Victor M. Alcoholic dementia. Can J Neurological Sci 1994;21 (suppl 2): 88-99.

3

REACHING A DIAGNOSIS AND ASSESSMENT

3.1

TAKING A HISTORY

Successful history taking requires use of skills derived from the realms of both science (fact-finding) and art (empathy). A thorough and sensitive history will act as the foundation for a good therapeutic relationship between patient, family and professionals.

When presented with a patient who may have a dementing illness, the first step must always be to take a full history. This should:

- establish the presence or absence of symptoms of organic brain disease
- describe premorbid functional ability and behaviour
- record past and present general medical status and medication.

To compensate for the memory impairment and lack of awareness (anosognosia) that often characterises even the most mildly demented patient, it is essential to gather information from both the patient and a reliable informant, ideally a close relative or friend. Both should be given a chance to tell their story out of earshot of the other.

A structured interview schedule covering the essential elements of the history forms the first two parts of the CAMDEX (Cambridge Examination for Mental Disorders of the Elderly). The Informant Questionnaire on Cognitive Decline in the Elderly (IQCODE) may be used to document an informant's report of changes in the everyday cognitive function of an elderly person compared with 10 years ago.

Conducting the Interview

- The first few minutes are crucial, as initial impressions will greatly influence the nature of the subsequent doctor-patient relationship. Light conversation about the weather or how the patient got to the clinic will act as an icebreaker and help to start building a rapport.

- Are there unnecessary distractions? Is the patient's hearing and vision optimised? Is the seating comfortable?

- The order in which material is collected needs to be flexible and adaptive. Too rigid a system may inhibit the patient, who may feel the interviewer is not really listening to what they want to say. If the patient is at ease and feels more in command of the situation, they will be less defensive and more likely to divulge all relevant information.

- Adequate time must be allowed for the interview and sometimes it will be best conducted over more than one session. Patience is necessary if all relevant information is to be adequately discussed. Allowing the patient a chance to ask questions may provide insights not otherwise forthcoming.

- Whilst taking the history, attention should also be given to the non-verbal communication of the patient. Is there good eye contact? Does his demeanour suggest depression or anxiety? Is he dressed and groomed appropriately?

- Specific attention should be given to the caregivers' emotional and physical state. How much practical care and supervision do they undertake? How much strain are they under? How much do they understand about the nature of the patient's condition? What are their needs and expectations for the future?

- Reviewing all available previous medical records is always instructive.

- A structured telephone interview to gather information about a patient after their death is also available. This enables retrospective clinical diagnosis of the presence and type of dementia.

Table. *Elements of the Medical History*

Presenting symptoms

Onset - gradual or acute
Subsequent course
Any remissions or exacerbations
Duration

Other symptoms of organic brain disturbance
(Record specific examples of problems experienced)

Memory impairment (recent and remote)
Language difficulties (poor conversational ability, misunderstanding, repetition)
Reading, writing, calculation problems
Attention problems
Apraxia, agnosia
Poor judgement

Psychiatric/behavioural symptoms

Hallucinations or delusions
Depression
Anxiety
Aggression
Wandering
Loss of confidence
Clinging/shadowing
Sleep disturbance

Ability to carry out day to day activities

Personal care (bathing, grooming, dressing continence)
Mobility
Shopping

Handling finances
Responsibility/compliance with medication
Using telephone
Travelling
Driving

Past and present medical status

Significant medical condition (especially neurological and systemic disorders)
History of head injury
History of depression or other psychiatric illness
Vascular risk factors (hypertension, diabetes, cardiac disease, hypercholesterolaemia)

Current medication

What has been prescribed to the patient?
What is the patient actually taking (including over-the-counter medication?)
What effects (good and bad) have current drugs?

Family history

Draw a family tree, showing age and present health or cause of death. Note particularly:
Dementia, 'senility', or admission to institution
Parkinson's disease
Down's syndrome
Stroke
Heart disease
Hypertension
Depression or other psychiatric disease

Education and occupational history

Age when left school
Any higher education
Nature of job when working
Any problems at work
Circumstances of retirement

Past and present alcohol intake

Smoking habit

Previous personality and coping ability (and any recent change)

- Interests and hobbies
- Energy and drive
- Concern for others
- Relationships with family and friends
- Social competence

Social background

- Family structure
- Current social contacts
- Emotional and physical demands on carers and their coping abilities
- Involvement of formal community support services
- Financial circumstances

FURTHER READING AND REFERENCES

CAMDEX - The Cambridge Examination for Mental Disorders of the Elderly. Cambridge University Press.

Jorm AF, Jacomb PA. An Informant Questionnaire on Cognitive decline in the Elderly (IQCODE): socio-demographic correlates, reliability, validity and some norms. Psychological Medicine 1989; 19: 1015-22.

Davis PB, White H, Price JL, et al. Retrospective postmortem dementia assessment: validation of a new clinical interview to assist neuropathologic study. Arch Neurol 1991; 48: 613-7.

3.2

FORMAL ASSESSMENT - Principles and Approach

Formal assessment can establish strengths and weaknesses of a variety of functions relative to a standardised, norm-referenced scoring system. It is important to plan the assessment approach to be used according to the specific purposes for which assessment is undertaken.

- Establishing the presence of cognitive deficits can usually be undertaken by the selection of a single screening scale or set of procedures, which can be administered effectively by any suitably trained professional..

- Objective assessment will be especially useful in cases of mild to moderate dementia, before the diagnosis is clinically obvious to even an untrained observer.

- Establishing specific patterns of cognitive deficits (and intact functioning) requires that screening procedures are supplemented by more specific tests, ideally administered by psychologists or neuropsychologists.

- Differential diagnosis of depression and dementia requires a further sophistication and the availability of specific test materials developed for such purposes.

- Formal assessment of the impact on carers of living with and looking after a person with dementia may be undertaken using self-completed or interview-administered questionnaires and rating scales.

- Assessment with a view to care management may require the use of behavioural checklists and tasks identifying strengths and weaknesses in functional independence, self-care and safety.

- Recording response to drug interventions requires repeated use of an appropriate measure of cognition, behaviour, ADL and global function, as well as a measure of the impact on caregivers.

Considerations In Test Administration

- Tests and test procedures must be acceptable to the person being tested, with no content that belittles their adult status. The tester will need to spend some time in explanation of the purpose of specific tests, and should be competent to answer queries regarding their usefulness and acceptability.

- Consent to the assessment procedure must be obtained, again following an explanation and justification of the usefulness of objective tests, with reassuring emphasis that such tests highlight strengths as well as weaknesses.

- The duration of assessment should be limited in accordance with the patient's tolerance of procedures, which will be influenced by degree of dementia and physical frailty. 15-20 minutes may be a suitable duration of assessment for many, although those with good concentration may cope well with assessments up to 45-60 minutes. A person in the early stages of a dementing illness will be able to perform a variety of tests in a shorter period than those with more advanced dementia. This is probably due to a relative preservation of cognitive speed and information-processing capacity. It has the advantage that more assessment information is obtainable in a shorter time period.

- Realistic reassurance should be given to the person being tested regarding their performance, with an acknowledgement of the demanding nature of some test materials. Feedback should be phrased positively, with an emphasis on observations of strengths during testing, i.e. preserved cognitive functions where these are observed. People should be reassured that the tests are not designed to give 'pass or fail' scores, and they should be given an opportunity to make their own observations on their performance at the end of testing.

- Sensory and physical limitations should be accommodated as much as possible, by the provision of adequate lighting, additional specialist earphone amplifiers, suitable seating etc.

Considerations In Test Selection

- Repeat assessment on at least two occasions should be considered to provide the best chance of obtaining reliable information, and tests should therefore be selected which can be administered on more than one occasion with unchanged validity.

- Standardised tests that have been developed and tested to high demands of reliability and validity should be selected over non-standardised tests. Assessment tools that provide age-referenced norms for a range of older age-groups should be selected where possible.

- Brief cognitive screening procedures should be included amongst other assessments, as long term monitoring is ideally achieved by repeat administration of such measures.

- Detailed, function-specific neuropsychological tests should always be administered in addition to screening tests in suspected early dementia. In mild dementia, screening tests fail to reliably identify minimal cognitive impairment in individuals of high pre-morbid intellectual functioning. Even in mild to moderate AD, different sub-types exist which present with varied patterns on tests of specific cognitive functions.

- Most screening tests are designed for detecting cortical rather than subcortical deficits and should be supplemented by a simple measure of executive function.

- When possible, assessment should be made of pre-morbid intellectual status, to assist in the satisfactory interpretation of other test scores.

- Tests must be appropriately selected to take account of limitations imposed by deficits such as language impairment and dyspraxia. For example, recognition memory tests may reduce the demand on expressive language, normally required in recall-memory tests.

Considerations In Test Interpretation

- In brief cognitive screening procedures in particular, the role of pre-morbid intellectual status, education, age, sensory impairments and co-morbidity should all be borne in mind when interpreting test scores.

- Observations of the person's concentration, co-operation, anxiety and motivation during assessment should be carefully weighed against performance. Are results a valid reflection of the person's true abilities?

- Attitude, interest and curiosity regarding the purpose of testing and its outcome all provide valuable, observational information about the person's status.

- Have cognitive deficits been observed on repeat assessment? Longitudinal follow up increases the accuracy of diagnosis, particularly in mild dementia.

- It must always be remembered that cognitive test results cannot be diagnostic on their own. Their usefulness lies in the additional information such test results bring to a range of other investigations, including clinical interview, detailed history obtained from a reliable informant, medical examination and appropriate investigations.

3.3

COGNITIVE ASSESSMENT - *Some Available Measures*

There is a very wide choice of assessment measures suitable for use with dementing patients and choice will be governed by the purpose of the examination and the time available, as well as personal preference and experience.

- **Mini Mental State Examination (MMSE).** *(Folstein MF et al. J Psychiatry Research 1975; 12: 189-198)* This is the most widely used and most investigated short screening test of cognitive impairment. It takes 5-10 minutes to complete. The 30 questions cover orientation, registration and recall, attention and calculation, writing and copying a simple geometric design. It is insensitive to frontal lobe impairment and has floor effects in severe dementia. A score of less than 24 best discriminates impairment from normality, though performance is influenced by age and past education.. The answers to individual questions can often be more informative than the overall score.

- **Cambridge Cognitive Examination (CAMCOG).** *(Roth M et al. Br J Psychiatry 1986; 149: 698-709).* This is the cognitive subsection of the CAMDEX and is broadly an expanded version of the MMSE, with additional sections measuring perception and remote memory. The revised version also contains additional measures of executive function. It takes 20-30 minutes to administer and requires specific test materials. It is less prone to ceiling effects than the MMSE and may therefore be more useful in mildly impaired patients.

- **Abbreviated Memory Test (AMT).** *(Qureshi KN, Hodkinson HM. Age Ageing 1974; 3: 152-157).* This is a brief 10-item test, derived from the longer Blessed Information-Memory-Concentration test. It is widely used in hospitals in the UK, but is only useful as a crude screening test for major impairment. A score of 6/10 or less indicates significant pathology.

- **Addenbrooke's Cognitive Examination (ACE).** *(Mathuranath PS, et al. Neurology 2000; 55: 1613-20)* This is a bedside schedule that incorporates the MMSE, but expands tests of memory, language and visuospatial function and adds tests of verbal fluency.

- **Mattis Dementia Rating Scale (DRS).** *(Mattis S. In Bellack R and Karasu B (eds). Geriatric Psychiatry. New York, Grune and Stratton 1976, 77-101)* This provides a global measure of dementia severity and is made up of five subscales (attention, initiation, construction, conceptualisation, memory). It takes 30-40 minutes, but is easy to administer and score, yielding a total ranging from 0 to 144 (perfect). It tends not to suffer from floor or ceiling effects.

- **Alzheimer's Disease Assessment Scale – Cognitive Subscale (ADAS-Cog).** *(Rosen WG et al, Amer J Psychiatry 1984; 141: 1356-1364).* This is a well-validated measure, widely used in clinical trials to evaluate severity of cognitive deficits and their response to drug treatment. It takes 20-30 minutes to complete and consists of a short battery of cognitive tests, including word recall, naming, commands, constructional and ideational praxis, orientation, word recognition, spoken language and comprehension, word-finding and recall of test instructions. Together these yield a total score between 0 (no impairment) and 70. Validated versions are available in most major European languages. The associated rating scale of non-cognitive symptoms is now little used.

- **Severe Impairment Battery (SIB).** *(Panisset M, et al. Severe Impairment Battery. A neuropsychological test for* *severly demented patients. Arch Neurol 1994; 51:41-6).* A simple assessment for people with moderate or severe dementia, developed to avoid the common problem of floor effects with most other cognitive measures. Nine different cognitive domains are assessed, relying on single word or one step commands, as well as gestures and behaviour. The scores range from 0 to 100.

- **Clifton Assessment Procedures for the Elderly (CAPE).** *(Pattie AH, Gilleard CJ. Br J Psychiatry 1978; 133: 457-460).* This consists of 3 parts - a 12 question information/orientation test, a behaviour rating scale (derived from the Stockton Geriatric Rating scale) and a psychomotor task, the Gibson Spiral Maze. Each part can also be used independently. It was originally designed for use with institutionalised patients and is most useful for providing guidance about suitable placement.

- **Syndrom Kurztest (SKT)** *(Overall JE, Schaltenbrand R. J Geriatr Psychiatry Neurol 1992; 5: 220-227)* This brief battery of cognitive tests, assessing attention and memory has been used extensively in clinical trials in dementia in German-speaking countries.The timebased scoring means that it takes 10-15 minutes to administer in all patients.

- **Clock Drawing** *(Shulman K et al. Int J Geriatr Psychiatry 1986; 1; 135-140).* Subjects are presented with a circle and asked to insert the numbers of a clock face and then place the hands at five to two. It is quick, simple, acceptable and informative, primarily testing visuoconstructional ability and executive function. The CLOX test has a detailed 15 point scoring system and requires the subject to free draw and copy a clock face, the difference in scores of the two versions being a measure of dysexecutive function (*Royall DR et al. J Neurology Neurosurg Psychiatry 1996; 64: 588-694*)

- **Hopkins Verbal Learning Test (HVLT).** *(Brandt J. Clin Neuropsychologist 1991; 5: 125-142).* A well validated measure of episodic memory, sensitive to early AD. A 12-item word list is presented and a total recall score and learning index calculated. A recognition test follows, with 12 original and 12 distractor words presented and a discrimination index (true positive vs. false positive) is calculated.

- **Story Recall**. A short story containing 15-25 defined elements is read to the subject, who then recalls the story in as much detail as possible. Both immediate and delayed recall (after 10-15 minutes) are tested. Delayed recall is especially sensitive to AD and other episodic memory disorders and correlates well with everyday memory difficulty.

- **Boston Naming Test** *(Kaplan E, et al. Philadelphia, Lea and Febiger, 1983).* The subject is required to name up to 60 line-drawings of objects, graded from very familiar to obscure. This measures word finding and semantic memory ability.

- **Verbal fluency** *(Morris JC, et al. Neurology 1999; 39: 1159-1165).* The subject must name as many animals (category fluency) as possible in 1 minute (category fluency). Alternatively they are asked to list as many words beginning with each of the letters 'FAS', with 1 minute allowed per letter (letter fluency). This simple test is sensitive to executive dysfunction and semantic memory impairment.

- **Computer-based neuropsychological test batteries** *(e.g. **CANTAB**; Morris et al. In Stahl S, Iversen S, Goodman E (eds). Cognitive Neurochemistry. Oxford, Oxford University Press 1987, 21-36 and **CDR**, Simpson PM et al. Int J geriatr psychiatry 1991; 6: 95-102)* are mainly used in research settings and are sensitive to small changes in performance and allow detailed assessment of attention and motor responses.

Table *Simple bedside tests of specific cognitive deficits*

Orientation	Time Place Person
Attention	Serial seven's subtraction Months of the year backwards
Abstraction	Proverb interpretation Cognitive estimates Similarities
Memory/Learning	Immediate (digit span) Remote (personal history, past events) Verbal memory (story repetition, names learning) Visual memory (object recall, reproducing designs)
Language	Comprehension (following complex commands) Naming (body parts, colours) Verbal fluency (animals, letters of alphabet) Reading and writing
Constructional skill	Clock drawing, copying designs (cube, intersecting pentagons)
Apraxia	Miming activities
Agnosia	Finger identification

3.4

NEUROPSYCHIATRIC ASSESSMENTS- *Some Available Measures*

Assessment of neuropsychiatric symptoms and behavioural disturbance is an important part of the comprehensive evaluation of the person with dementia. They are important sources of distress to carers as well as to patients and a common reason for institutionalisation.

Table. *Common neuropsychiatric symptoms in dementia*

Abnormal eating behaviours
Affective disorders/mood disturbances
Agitation
Anxiety
Apathy
Compulsive/ritualistic behaviours
Delusions
Demanding/critical behaviour
Disinhibition
Fearfulness
Hallucinations
Irritability
Illusions
Incontinence
Kluver-Bucy syndrome
Misidentifications
Personality change
Phobia
Restlessness
Shouting/screaming
Rage/violence
Sleep-wake disturbances
Sexual behaviours
Sundowning
Wandering

- **Neuropsychiatric Inventory (NPI)** *(Cummings JL, et al. Neurology 1994; 44: 2308-14).* This measure has become the most commonly used rating scale of psychopathology in dementia. 12 behavioural disturbances are assessed in a standardised interview with a carer, using a screening strategy to cut down on time of administration. The behavioural areas explored are delusions, hallucinations, agitation, depression, anxiety, euphoria, apathy, disinhibition, irritability, aberrant motor behaviour, night-time behaviours and appetite and eating disorders. Severity and frequency are independently assessed, with a maximum possible score of 144. The distress caused to carers by each behaviour can also be rated.

- **BEHAVE-AD** *(Reisberg B, et al. J Clin Psychiatry 1987; 48 (suppl 5): 9-15).* This was the first rating scale of behaviour in Alzheimer's disease, designed to measure symptomatology at different stages of the disease and in response to drug intervention. The 25 questions cover paranoid and delusional ideation, hallucinations, activity disturbances, aggressiveness, diurnal rhythm disturbances, affective disturbance and anxieties and phobias. The clinician is also required to rate how troubling the symptoms are to the carer or dangerous to the patient.

- **Behavioural Rating Scale for Dementia** *(Tariot PN, et al. Am J Psychiatry 1995; 152:1349-1357)* The frequency of each of 51 symptoms is rated by semi-structured interview with a carer. The symptoms are grouped under 8 factors, depression, psychosis, defective self-regulation, irritability/agitation, vegetative features, apathy, aggression and affective lability.

- **Nurse's Observation Scale for Geriatric Patients (NOSGER)** *(Spiegel R, et al. J Am Geriatr Soc 1991; 39: 339-47)* This 30 item assessment of behaviour and functioning in institutionalised and community-living elderly patients can be completed by nursing staff or lay people. Each item is rated on the basis of frequency by direct observation. Questions that may upset some relatives because of their negative connotations were not included.

Geriatric Depression Scale (*Yesavage JA, et al. J Psychiatric Res 1983; 17: 37-49).* This simple self-administered or interview-administered scale was designed specifically for rating depression in elderly people. A 30, 15 and 4-item version exist, each question having a yes/no answer, with scoring dependent on the answer given. Validity in the presence of Alzheimer's disease is less certain (Burke WJ, et al J Am Geriatr Soc 1989; 37: 856-60)

- **Cornell Scale for Depression in Dementia** *(Alexopoulos GS, et al. Biol Psychiatry 1988; 23: 271-84).* A 19-item clinician-rated scale based on interview with patient and carer and designed to diagnose depression in people with dementia.

- **Dementia Mood Assessment Scale** *(Sunderland T, et al. Am J Psychiatry 1988; 145: 955-9).* This 24-item scale (17 depression items and 7 dementia severity items) measures mood in people with mild to moderate dementia. A trained clinician completes the assessment by semi-structured interview and observation.

- **Rating Scale for Aggressive Behaviour in the Elderly (RAGE).** *(Patel V, Hope RA. Psychological Med 1992; 22: 211-21)* A 21-item assessment of aggressive behaviour in psychogeriatric inpatients, designed to be completed in a few minutes by nursing staff.

- **Cohen-Mansfield Agitation Inventory (CMAI).** *(Cohen-Mansfield J. J Am Geriatr Soc 1986; 34: 722-7)* Trained observers rate specific behavioural disturbances in people with dementia. The original 29-item version uses a 7-point frequency scale for each behaviour, but there are other shorter versions available (e.g. Brief Agitation Rating Scale. *Finkel SI et al. J Am Geriatr Soc 1993; 41: 50-2)*

3.5

ACTIVITIES OF DAILY LIVING ASSESSMENTS - *Some Available Measures*

Impairment of activities of daily living (ADL) is an integral part of dementia and is a major determinant of need for care. Preservation of ADL is an important aim of management. Loss of instrumental ADL precedes loss of basic ADL and there is a close association between progressive loss of functional ability and cognitve skills. It is highly influenced by gender and culture.
Assessment of ADL can be by direct observation or by carer rating using a standardised questionnaire.

- **Progressive Deterioration Scale** *(DeJong et al, Clin Ther 1989; 11: 545-54)*. Whilst has been presented as a QOL measure, this carer-completed measure is more appropriately considered to be an assessment of aspects of IADL in people with AD. There are 29 items yielding a score ranging from 0 to 100.

- **Bristol Activities of Daily Living Scale** *(Bucks et al. Age Ageing 1995; 25: 113-20.)* This 20-item questionnaire was developed for community-living people with dementia, with items selected on basis of carer feedback. It can be self-completed by carers or administered by interview and assesses both instrumental and basic ADL.

- **Disabilty Assessment for Dementia (DAD)** *(Gelinas I, et al. Am J Occup Therapy 1999; 53: 471-81)* Developed for use with people with dementia living in the community, this has been widely used in recent clinical trials to measure change in ADL and IADL. Each of 40 items in ten areas are assessed, with separate attention given to the areas of initiation, planning/organisation and effective performance.

- **Nurses Observation scale for Geriatric patients (NOSGER)** *Spiegel et al J Am Geriatr Soc 1991; 39: 339-47)* This assesses memory, mood and behaviour as well as ADL and IADL. Nurses rate each of the 30 items on the basis of frequency by direct observation.

- **Alzheimer's Disease Functional Assessment and Change Scale (ADFACS)** *(Galasko D, et al. Alz Dis Assoc Disord 1997; 11(suppl 2): S33-9).* This measure was designed to measure ADL in clinical trials and has been shown to be sensitive to change over 12 months. Based on carer interview, rating is made of 10 IADL items (each rated on a 5 point scale, including not assessable) and 7 basic ADL items (rated on a 6 point scale).

- **Functional Performance Measure (FPM)** *(Carswell A, et al. Can J Occup Therapy 1995; 62: 62-9).* This observational outcome measure was developed for people with AD and rates 39 items of ADL and IADL on motor performance, context, attention, perception, concentration, processing, planning and quality of performance.

- **Instrumental Activities of Daily Living (IADL)** *(Lawton M, Brody E. Gerontologist 1969; 9:179-86.)* This is one of the first measures of more complex ADL activities and is combined with the Physical Self-Maintenance Scale of basic ADL.

- **Interview for Deterioration in Daily Living Activities in dementia (IDDD)** *(Teunisse S, et al. Arch Neurol 1991; 48: 274-77)* This 33-item structured interview of carers includes self-care ADL and IADL items. Each item is rated on a 3-point scale of frequency of assistance, with total ranging from 33 to 99 (most severe).

3.6

QUALITY OF LIFE, GLOBAL ASSESSMENT AND DEMENTIA STAGING - *Some Available Measures*

QUALITY OF LIFE MEASURES

Despite the availability of a large number of quality of life (QOL) instruments, there is no 'gold standard'. Assessment of people with dementia is especially problematic and there is no consensus about the relative merits of patient completion (problematic for those with moderate and severe dementia) versus carer completion (that may not reflect patients' true experience). Some so-called QOL instruments actually measure quality of care. Potentially useful QOL instruments are:

- **Community Dementia QOL Profile (CDQLP).** (Salek MS, et al. Pharm World Sci 1996; 18: 5 suppl A): 6). This is a 33-item, dementia-specific instrument completed by the carer, acting as proxy to record the patient's QOL and also measuring their own QOL and burden. The psychometric properties of the instrument have been tested thoroughly.

- **Quality of Life-AD (QOL-AD)** *(Logsdon RG. Gerontologist 1996; 36 (special issue 1): 278.)* Both patient and carer rate the patient on each of 13 items (physical health, energy, mood, living situation, memory, family, marriage, friends, chores, fun, money, self and life as a whole) on a 4-point scale (from poor to excellent). A composite score is calculated that weights the patient rating more heavily than that of the carer.

- **Dementia QOL (DQOL)** *(Brod M. Gerontologist 1996; 36 (special issue 1): 257).* This 56-item measure (covering physical functioning, daily activities, discretionary activities, mobility, social wellbeing, interaction capacity, bodily wellbeing, psychological well being, sense of aesthetics and overall QOL) is designed for direct respondent assessment. It is brief and preliminary reliability and validity are established.

- **Blau QOL Scale** *(Blau TH. Prof Psychol 1977; 11: 464-73).* Aspects of QOL are rated on visual analogue scales by the patient, or a proxy. For use in clinical trials, the original 10 areas of interest were reduced to 7 (eating, sleeping, social contact, eating, loving, environment and self-acceptance).

- **Schedule for Evaluation of Individual Quality of Life (SEIQOL).** *(Coen R, et al. Irish J Psychol 1993; 14: 154-63).* Patients nominate the five areas of most importance for their QOL and rate their level of functioning and the relative importance of each. The assessment is time consuming and the analysis is complex. The approach is only appropriate for those with mild dementia.

GLOBAL MEASURES

An alternative approach to measuring the overall impact of dementia on the patient is to assess 'global function'. This is widely used as an outcome measure in clinical trials of anti-dementia drugs and is a requirement of regulatory authorities.

- **Clinician Interview Based Impression Of Severity/Change (CIBIS/CIBIC).** *Knopman DS, et al. Neurol 1994; 44: 2315-21*). An experienced clinician undertakes a thorough interview with the patient examining all available evidence and taking all factors into account at baseline (CIBIS). Subsequent assessments rate overall change from baseline on a 7-point scale, as no change, or minimal, moderate or marked improvement or worsening. It is usual also to interview the carer and the assessments are then termed CIBIS-plus and CIBIC-plus. In some versions of the CIBIS/CIBIC, the interview is semi-structured to ensure coverage of specific domains.

- **Clinical Global Impression Of Change (CGIC).** *(Schneider L, et al. Alz Dis Assoc Disord 1997; 11 (suppl 2): 322-32)* This rating incorporates information from both patient and carer and uses an unstructured interview format that covers the domains of memory, language, orientation, praxis, mood, behaviour and ADL. The rater can choose his own assessments for each domain. The final rating is made on a 7-point scale.

DEMENTIA STAGING INSTRUMENTS

Formal staging measures are useful for describing dementia severity in individual patients and for selecting patient groups, but are not very sensitive to change.

- **Clinical Dementia Rating (CDR)** *(Berg L. Psychopharmacol Bull 1988; 24: 637-9).* Ratings of 0 (normal), 0.5 (questionable), 1 (mild), 2 (moderate) or 3 (severe) are made of 6 domains. These are memory, orientation, judgement and problem solving, community affairs, home and hobbies and personal care. Ratings are based on all available evidence and patient/carer interview. An algorithm that weights the memory component is used to give an overall rating from 0 to 3 (with scores of 4 for profound and 5 for terminal also available). Alternatively the individual scores of each domain are summed to give the sum of boxes (CDR-SB), ranging from 0 to 18.

- **Global Deterioration Scale (GDS)** *(Reisberg B, et al. Am J Psychiatry 1982; 139: 1136-9).* This is a 7-point staging measure, ranging from stage 1 (normal) to stage 7 (severe dementia). Stage 3 would now be MCI and stage 4 is mild dementia. The patient is placed into the stage of highest incapacity.

3.7

CARER ASSESSMENTS - *Some Available Measures*

There is growing interest in assessing the impact of caring for a person with dementia on those providing care. Psychological and physical burden can be measured, as well as the time taken up with caring.

- **Relatives' Stress Scale** *(Greene JG, et al. Age Ageing 1982; 11: 121-6).* This 15 item scale measures personal distress, degree of life upset and negative feelings to the patient in the relatives of people with dementia. Each item is scored on a 5 point scale. It takes about 5-10 minutes to complete. The Relative's Stress Scale was developed alongside the Behavioural and Mood Disturbance Scale for use with people with dementia living at home.

- **General Health Questionnaire (GHQ)** *(Goldberg DP, Williams P. Windsor, NFER-NELSON 1988).* This has been widely used as a measure of psychological distress and psychiatric morbidity in carers, though it was designed for detecting psychiatric disorder in the general adult population in the community. There are versions including 12, 28, 30 and 60 questions (taking from 5 to 20 minutes to complete).

- **Screen For Caregiver Burden (SCB)** *(Vitaliano PP, Gerontologist 1991; 31: 76-83)* A 25-item scale measuring perceived burden (both subjective and objective) of caring for a person with dementia.

- **Carer Strain Scale** *(Gilleard CJ. Living with dementia:community care of the elderly mentally infirm. Beckenham, Croom Helm 1984)* This rates the frequency of 13 potential problems on a 3-point scale: never present, sometimes present, or present a great deal of the time. The items assessed include safety, embarrassment, sleep, coping, depression, worry, household routine, frustration, enjoyment of role, holidays, finance, health and demands for attention. A 34-item problem checklist rating aspects of behaviour of the person with dementia accompanies the strain scale.

- **Caregiver Activity Survey (CAS).** *(Davis KL, et al. Int J Geriatr Psychiatry 1997; 12: 978-88).* This is a brief measure that asks carers to estimate the amount of time spent over 24 hours looking after a person with dementia. The areas assessed include communication, using transportation, dressing, eating, looking after self-appearance and need for supervision.

- **Caregiver Hassles Scale** *(Kinney JM, Stephens MAP. Gerontologist 1989; 29: 328-332).* This was developed to record the impact of caregiving on day-to-day life of carers. There are 42 items related to basic ADL, instrumental ADL, cognition, behaviour and the carer's support network.

- **Burden Interview** *(Zarit SH, et al. Gerontologist 1980; 20: 649-55)* This 29 item interview assesses the feelings of burden of carers when caring for an elderly person with dementia. It was one of the first measures to highlight their burden and needs.

- **Caregiver Strain Index** *(Robinson B. Validation of a caregiver strain index. J Gerontol 1983; 38: 344-8)* The original version assesses presence or absence of 13 factors that may be a source of strain when caring for a person with dementia. A modified version uses a 4 point scale to answer each question and standardises the overall score to range from 0 (no burden) to 100.

REFERENCES AND FURTHER READING

Bayer AJ, Synan CA. Functional assessment scales. In: Pathy MSJ (ed). Principles and Practice of Geriatric Medicine. Chichester, John Wiley 1998.

Burns A, Lawlor B, Craig S. Assessment Scales in Old Age Psychiatry. London, Martin Dunitz 1999

Lezak MD. Neuropsychological Assessment. New York, Oxford University Press, 1983.

Hodges JR. Cognitive Assessment for Clinicians. Oxford, Oxford University Press 1994.

Howard K, Rockwood K. Quality of life in Alzheimer's disease: a review. Dementia 1995; 6: 113-6.

Shulman KI, Feinstein A. Quick Cognitive Screening for Clinicians. London, Martin Dunitz 2003

Hart S, Semple JM. Neuropsychology and the Dementias. London: Taylor & Francis, 1990.

Walker MD, Salek SS, Bayer AJ. A review of quality of life iin Alzheimer's disease. Pharmacoeconomics 1998; 14: 499-530.

3.8

MEDICAL EXAMINATION

The medical examination of the demented patient may

- help to elucidate the cause of the illness
- identify physical consequences of the condition
- identify coexisting morbidities

As most patients will be elderly, multiple pathology is almost inevitable and trying to attribute all abnormalities to a single diagnosis will rarely be possible.

General examination.

- Look for general evidence of poor hygiene and self neglect (uncut toe nails, faeces under the fingernails, matted hair). Skin problems may range from age-related dryness and flaking to more serious pressure sores or infestations.

- Vitamin deficiencies often manifest themselves by changes in the skin and mucous membranes. Bruising may be caused by ascorbic acid deficiency, but the examiner should also be alert to the possibility of physical abuse.

- Use a low reading thermometer if there is a possibility of hypothermia

- Note any signs of dehydration.

Cardio-respiratory system.

- Patients with vascular dementia especially are likely to have evidence of heart disease and hypertension. Identification of cardiac dysrhythmias, especially atrial fibrillation and sustained bradycardia, is important.

- Blood pressure should be measured standing as well as sitting. Palpation of the apex beat to estimate cardiac size is unreliable. Auscultation may reveal added heart sounds, murmurs or bruits indicating a need for further investigation. Carotid bruits might suggest carotid stenosis and a source of emboli in VaD.

- Tachypnoea may alert the examiner to significant cardiac, chest, or metabolic disease.

Gastrointestinal system.

- Examination should start at the mouth, with careful inspection of teeth and dentures and of the oral cavity. Angular stomatitis may suggest poorly fitting dentures, candidiasis or vitamin B deficiency. Assessment of nutritional status is important in all patients and recording the weight is a useful baseline measure in even the well nourished.

- Hepatomegaly and other stigmata of liver disease might suggest alcohol-related problems, hepatic encephalopathy or malignancy.

- Rectal examination is mandatory in anyone reporting altered bowel habit or faecal incontinence (most often due to impaction and overflow). The nose is usually the most reliable detector of incontinence.

Central Nervous System

- Focal neurological signs indicate focal pathology. They are usually to be found in vascular dementia, but are rare in degenerative dementia, at least until late in the disease.

Loss of muscle bulk is more often due to lack of use rather than denervation. Extensor plantar responses may be associated with cervical spondylosis rather than cortical disease. Muscle fasiculation may suggest motor neurone disease associated with FTD. Gegenhalten must be distinguished from the increased tone associated with pyramidal or extrapyramidal disease.

- Primitive reflexes (e.g. palmo-mental, grasp, pout, rooting, sucking) are common in all most forms of dementia, though not always easy to elicit.

- Involuntary movements may be associated with Huntington's disease and Wilson's disease, but much more often are due to anti-Parkinsonian or neuroleptic drugs. Sudden onset of hemichorea is likely to be due to stroke. A wandering dystonic arm (alien limb) may suggest corticobasal degeneration. Parkinsonian tremor must be distinguished from benign essential tremor. Myoclonus is seen in CJD, Huntington's disease and early onset AD.

- Is there evidence of dysarthria?

Eyes and ears

- Examination of the eye may identify hemianopia or visual inattention (suggesting vascular disease), or incidental cataract or glaucoma. Is the patient wearing the appropriate spectacles and are the lenses clean?

- Are eye movements full, or is there a gaze palsy suggesting PSP? Is there nystagmus?

- Fundoscopy may reveal hypertensive or diabetic retinopathy, or rarely papilloedema associated with a space-occupying lesion.

- Examination of the ears for wax is essential in any patient with hearing loss. If a hearing aid is used, it is being worn, in the correct ear, are the batteries working and is the ear mould clean?

Gait

- Always watch the patient walking. Is there evidence of ataxia, hemiplegia, 'marche a petis pas' (short stepped gait with upright posture and good arm swing suggestive of vascular disease or frontal lobe impairment), or Parkinsonism? Can the patient easily get up unaided from a chair? Backward leaning is especially common after a period of bedrest. Are any walking aids being used correctly? Does limited mobility indicate a need for chiropody? Is footwear appropriate?

Finally, whenever possible the medical, examination should also include the patient's immediate home environment. Is it well maintained or is there evidence of neglect? Are security, lighting and heating adequate? Are there empty bottles suggesting excessive alcohol intake? Is food being hoarded or is the kitchen bare? Are hearing aids, glasses and walking aids readily available?

FURTHER READING AND REFERENCES

Chen JY, Stern Y, Sano M, et al. Cumulative risk of developing extrapyramidal signs, psychosis, or myoclonus in the course of Alzheimer's disease. Arch Neurol 1991; 48: 1141-3.

Franssen EH, Reisberg B, Kluger A, Sinaiko E, et al. Cognitive independent neurologic symptoms in normal ageing and probable Alzheimer's disease. Arch Neurol 1991; 48: 148-54.

Galasko D, Yuen PFK, Klauber MR, et al. Neurological findings in Alzheimer's disease and normal ageing. Arch Neurol 1990; 47: 625-7.

Geldmacher DS, Whitehouse PJ. Evaluation of dementia. NEJM 1996; 335: 330-6.

3.9

NEUROIMAGING

Neuroimaging no longer merely fulfils the negative role of excluding 'treatable' conditions that mimic or cause dementia, but positively contributes to differential diagnosis and can provide useful prognostic information.

Depending on availability, computed tomography (CT), magnetic resonance imaging (MRI) and single photon emission computed tomography (SPECT) may all contribute to clinical care. Various other techniques are available in research centres.

Recent diagnostic guidelines suggest that at least one structural CT or MRI examination should be made over the course of a dementing illness to rule out space occupying or vascular lesions, and that SPECT (or PET) should be used in cases of significant diagnostic uncertainty. However, in practice it is not always possible to perform neuroimaging in every elderly patient with dementia. Indications for scanning have therefore been proposed:

- Focal CNS signs
- Recent onset of epileptic fits
- Recent head injury
- Any suspicion of intracranial tumour, including raised intracranial pressure, or evidence of a source for metastases outside the brain
- Any suspicion of NPH
- Any suspicion of stroke disease

- **Computed tomography (CT)** is probably the radiological investigation of choice in most patients with dementia, owing to its wide availability. It can show good detail of the brain structure and is especially useful in identifying dementia due to space occupying lesions, hydrocephalus or large cerebral infarcts. Smaller lacunar infarcts are less easily seen and absence of infarcts does not exclude the possibility of vascular dementia.

  Generalized and localized cortical atrophy is a common finding in older patients, not necessarily associated with clinically abnormal brain function. Some patients with AD will have a normal scan. Nevertheless, the presence of atrophy is useful supportive evidence of degenerative brain disease. In AD, there is generalized cortical atrophy, whereas frontal atrophy may suggest FTD. Marked atrophy of the caudate nuclei is seen in Huntington's disease. Serial CT measurement is particularly useful, but not often possible. Change in size of the lateral ventricles over a few months is a sensitive marker of AD.

- **Magnetic resonance imaging (MRI)** is less widely available, less convenient for patients and more expensive than CT. However, contrast sensitivity and spatial resolution is better, even without use of contrast agents and it does not suffer from bone artefacts. Evidence of generalized atrophy is no more diagnostically useful than with CT, but measuremont of the size of the hippocampus and entorhinal cortex plays an important role not only in diagnosis of AD, but also in identifying premorbid at risk patients (i.e. those with MCI).

  Smaller infarcts can be seen more clearly than with CT and MRI has the potential to detect focal signal abnormalities that may assist the clinical differentiation between AD and VaD. Severe temporal lobe atrophy, hyperintensities involving the hippocampal or insular cortex, and gyral hypointense bands are more frequently noted in AD. Basal ganglionic/thalamic hyperintense foci, thromboembolic infarctions, confluent white matter and irregular periventricular hyperintensities (leukoencephalopathy) are more common in VaD.

Leukoencephalopathy involving at least 25% of the total white matter must be present to diagnose small vessel cerebrovascular disease.

Several other imaging findings seem to be sensitive enough to serve as useful diagnostic criteria, such as focal frontal-temporal atrophy, for the diagnosis of FTD; elevated signal in the striatum bilaterally, for the diagnosis of sporadic CJD, or in the pulvinar bilaterally for the diagnosis of variant CJD.

Other magnetic resonance techniques include:

* **diffusion-weighted MR imaging (DWI)** measures the molecular mobility of water in tissue and shows an increase in diffusion values in selected regions of interest in AD and MCI patients compared to controls.

* **dynamic susceptibility contrast MR imaging (DSC MRI)** measures the rate at which blood is delivered to tissue.and can identify the characteristic bilateral temporo-parietal perfusion/metabolism defects also seen with SPECT/PET in AD patients.

* **functional MR (fMRI)** examination of declarative memory can serve as a functional medial-temporal *stress test", though significant technical problems remain to be solved.

* **MR spectroscopy (MRS)** can measure characteristic abnormalities associated with AD, such as decrease in N-acetyl aspartate (NAA) and an elevation in myoinositol (MI). It is suggested that the initial MRS change in the pathological progression of AD is an increase in MI. A decrease in NAA develops later in the disease.

Structural and functional MRI techniques have great potential in identifying patients at risk for AD, which will allow for very early treatment with drugs that slow or even halt progression.

- **Single photon emission computed tomography (SPECT)** allows regional cerebral blood flow to be visualized and quantified. In established AD there is a reduction of flow in frontal and temporo-parietal regions, though this finding is inconsistent in the early stage of the disease when diagnosis is most problematic. In FTD and PSP, SPECT shows diminished perfusion anteriorly. In vascular dementia, multiple focal deficits may be seen.

- **Positron emission tomography (PET)** has higher spatial resolution than SPECT and assesses regional cerebral metabolism. However, it is much more expensive and only available in a few centres. It is almost exclusively used as a research tool.

FURTHER READING AND REFERENCES

Frisoni GB, et al. Neuroimaging tools to rate regional atrophy, subcortical cerebrovascular disease, and regional cerebral blood flow and metabolism: consensus paper of the EADC. J Neurol Neurosurg Psychiatry 2003; 74: 1371-1381.

Lee BC, et al. Imaging of Alzheimer's disease. J Neuroimaging. 2003;13:199-214

Scheltens P, et al. Structural magnetic resonance imaging in the practical assessment of dementia beyond exclusion. Lancet Neurol. 2002; 1:13-21.

Thomas DL, et al. The measurement of diffusion and perfusion in biological systems using magnetic resonance imaging. Phys Med Biol. 2000;45:R97-138

Wahlund LO. Magnetic resonance imaging and computed tomography in Alzheimer's disease. Acta Neurol Scand Suppl. 1996;168:50-3.

Xanthakos S, et al. Magnetic resonance imaging of Alzheimer's disease. Prog Neuropsychopharmacol Biol Psychiatry. 1996;20:597-626

3.10

OTHER INVESTIGATIONS

How far to investigate a patient presenting with probable dementia will depend on the clinical features, concurrent medical conditions and ease of access to laboratory and radiological facilities. In practice, a balance must be struck between ensuring a treatable condition is not missed and unthinkingly submitting all patients to a regimen of sometimes upsetting and expensive investigations.

- A routine screening battery of **blood tests** will be indicated in most patients when first seen:
    - full blood court
    - urea and electrolytes
    - random blood glucose
    - liver function tests, including gamma-GT
    - thyroid function tests
    - vitamin B12 and folate

- A more extensive range of tests may be indicated in younger people with dementia and in those with atypical presentations or signs and evidence of systemic illness:
    - erythrocyte sedimentation rate (ESR), plasma viscosity and/or C-reactive protein (non-specific markers of infection or inflammation)
    - tumour markers (malignancy, paraneoplastic syndromes
    - serum calcium (hyperparathyroidism, metabolic bone disease)
    - syphilis serology
    - HIV

- autoantibodies (anti-nuclear factor for SLE, anti-soluble RNA antibody for scleroderma, anti-cardiolipin antibody for anti-phospholipid syndrome)
- serum copper and caeruloplasmin (for Wilson's disease). Heavy metal screen (for suspected poisoning)
- white cell arylsulphatase activity (for metachromatic leukodystrophy).

- **Genetic testing** is rarely indicated and should only be undertaken after appropriate counselling preferably in a specialist genetics clinic.Testing may be indicated in:
  - Suspected Huntington's disease (Huntington gene)
  - CADASIL (notch 3 gene mutation)
  - Familial AD (PS-1, PS-2, APP gene mutations)
  - Familial FTD (tau gene mutations)
  - Familal CJD (prion protein gene mutation)
  - Determination of apolipoprotein genotype is not diagnostically useful. Whilst prevalence of the e4 allele is significantly increased in AD, it is neither sufficient nor necessary for the diagnosis and is absent in 40% of patients with autopsy-confirmed AD.
- **Urinanalysis** and **mid stream urine (MSU)** sample should be tested in all patients with urinary symptoms, including those with incontinence and in those with possible delirium. Bacteriuria in the absence of relevant symptoms is unlikely to be significant and does not require treatment.

- An **electrocardiogram (ECG)** is desirable in any patient with possible vascular disease and in patients with a bradycardia or history of dysrhythmia who are being considered for anticholinesterase treatment. A 24 hour ECG may be useful in patients presenting with dementia associated with blackouts.

- A **chest X ray** may be valuable in those with cardio-respiratory symptoms and in previously heavy smokers

- An **echocardiogram and Doppler ultrasound** studies of the carotid arteries may indicate a source of emboli in patients with VaD

- An **electromyelogram (EMG)** in patients with dementia and muscle fasiculations may help to diagnose FTD associated with motor neurone disease.

- Biopsy for histopathological examination may be diagnostic in some conditions. **Muscle biopsy** will reveal 'ragged-red' changes in mitochondrial disorders. **Tonsillar biosy** can reveal the abnormal prion protein in variant CJD. **Cerebral biops**y is occasionally justified in patients with suspected cerenbral vasculitis.

- The **electroencephalogram (EEG)** is mainly useful in confirming the presence or absence of delirium, in which it is nearly always abnormal. In patients with dementia it is of less value.

  A normal EEG is consistent with a diagnosis of degenerative dementia, though diffuse slowing tends to develop in patients with moderate to severe AD. In FTD, the EEG is often normal even when symptoms are severe. In VaD, the tracing may be asymmetrical, with localised slow wave activity.

  Focal slowing may also be seen associated with space occupying lesions, such as a tumour, haematoma or abscess. In CJD, the EEG is characteristically abnormal with paroxysmal triphasic sharp waves and a slow background rhythm. The spike activity associated with epilepsy may also be useful diagnostically.

  Delay in components of the visual evoked potential has also been advocated as diagnostically useful in dementia (especially AD), but has not been widely adopted. EEG mapping is a specialist technique available in a few centres.

- **Cerebrospinal fluid (CSF)** examination may be diagnostically useful, though can be technically difficult in elderly patients with osteoarthritic spines and in uncooperative patients. It is especially valuable in patients with suspected infectious, inflammatory, autoimmune or demyelinating disease. In NPH it may help to predict response to surgery. Presence of the CSF 14-3-3 protein confirms the diagnosis of CJD.

  CSF markers of neurodegenerative disease are also attracting growing attention, as a means of increasing sensitivity of early diagnosis of AD. Elevated tau protein is associated with neural degeneration followed by disintegration of neurons. High phospho-tau is linked with hyperphosphorylation and is considered a more specific marker for AD, especially when associated with decreased level of beta amyloid. Evaluations of these three markers can support the diagnosis of AD and distinguish it from other dementias and vascular cognitive impairment. Detection of at least two positive "neurodegenerative markers" in the CSF has prognostic value in people with MCI, preceding manifestations of AD by 2-3 years.

FURTHER READING AND REFERENCES

Knopman DS, DeKosky ST, Cummings JL, et al. Practice Parameter: Diagnosis of Dementia (an Evidence-based Review). Neurology 2001; 56: 1143-53

Larson EB, Reifler BV, Sumi SM, et al. Diagnostic tests in the evaluation of dementia. A prospective study of 200 elderly outpatients. Arch Int Med 1986; 146: 1917-22.

Maruyama, M. et al. Cerebrospinal fluid amyloid beta (1-42) levels in mild cognitive impairment stage in Alzheimer's disease. Exp. Neurol 2001; 172: 433-6

Sjögren, M. et al. Both total and phosphorylated tau are increased in Alzheimer´s disease. J. Neurol. Neurosurg. Psychiatry 2001; 70: 624-630

Van Crevel H, Van Gool WA, Walstra GJM. Early diagnosis of dementia: which tests are indicated? What are their costs? J Neurology 1999; 246: 73-8.

4

MANAGEMENT

4.1

PRINCIPLES OF CARE – Personhood, Spiritual and Ethical Issues

Good management of demented patients requires considerable community-based resources, backed up by easily accessible hospital and residential facilities.

High standards of care provision are costly and demented patients will always be in competition with more immediately attractive and articulate groups, such as children and their parents and the young physically disabled. Those responsible for service provision should encourage open discussion of all the issues involved in providing care and decisions made should always be equitable and fair, rather than politically expedient.

Person-Centred Care

The concept of personhood and person-centred care has become central to provision of high quality dementia care.

- Person-centred care has its origins in the client-centred psychotherapy pioneered by Carl Rogers and was first applied in the field of dementia by Tom Kitwood. It brings together ideas and ways of working that emphasise communication and relationships.

- Seeing the person with dementia as an individual with rights and a need for sensitive interaction has also influenced and been influenced by developments such as reality orientation, validation, individual needs assessment and social role valorisation.

- Brooker has identified the four major elements of person-centred care as:

    - Valuing people with dementia and those who care for them.
    - Treating people as individuals.
    - Looking at the world from the perspective of the person with dementia
    - A positive social environment in which the person living with dementia can experience relative well-being.

- The technique of **Dementia Care Mapping** (DCM) is closely linked to person-centred care and is an attempt to help professionals to take the standpoint of the person with dementia when evaluating the quality of care, using a combination of empathy and observational skills.

- DCM provides staff with concrete feedback about how the people in their care are experiencing daily life, highlighting aspects of malignant social psychology and promoting a more positive approach. This information can be used to plan more person-centred care on an individual, group and organisational level.

When To Intervene?

Lack of effective curative treatment for most dementing illnesses does not mean that they are untreatable. Active treatment of troublesome symptoms and organisation of good quality care will favourably influence the outcome of all patients.

- Management plans should recognise patient's autonomy and focus on the goals of care, allowing everyone involved to become informed of options and of the consequences of possible treatment decisions.

- Aggressive management of all concurrent medical conditions is seldom justified. The decision to intervene will depend on the individual patient, but no one should ever be denied necessary care on the grounds of age or mental state.

- Management of terminal disease should aim to minimise suffering and maintain dignity. It would appear that the majority of older nursing home residents would only want comfort care and palliation in the event of advanced AD. Inappropriate prolongation of life by meddlesome intervention is morally as difficult to justify as active euthanasia.

- It is the moral responsibility of involved professionals to help the family to judiciously reach decisions to employ, withhold or withdraw life-sustaining treatments. Good care is based on good communication and positive action - or sometimes, inaction.

- Most expert guidelines favour the use of advance directives for those at risk of or those diagnosed with dementia. Earlier diagnosis has meant that the timely preparation of directives can be facilitated, though it is still only a small minority of people who wish to do so.

Involving The Family

It is impossible to treat the person with dementia in isolation from the family, particularly those providing immediate care.

- Family members often assess the quality of life of the individual with dementia more negatively than is justified. Sometimes there may be an apparent conflict of interests.

- Whilst the professional's primary responsibility is always to their patient, good management will usually require the patient and caregiver to be regarded as a partnership. Addressing carers' concerns will often result in a better long term outcome for the patient.

The Role Of Research

If treatment of dementia is to improve, then research is essential. Its unnecessary restriction must therefore be morally indefensible.

- Every individual with dementia should have the opportunity to take part in research. However, they also retain the right to refuse to cooperate, however seemingly illogical. Particular care must be taken when the professional undertaking research is also the person responsible for clinical care.

- Issues of consent and confidentiality must be respected and addressed and the limitations of proxy consent, both legally and practically, should be recognised. When informed consent from the person with dementia is not possible, consent from their legal representative (where available) or assent from a close relative is appropriate.

- Non-therapeutic research (without possible benefit to the individual involved) is especially difficult to justify in those unable to give their own fully informed consent.

FURTHER READING AND REFERENCES

Baldwin C, Hughes J, Hope T, et al. Ethics and dementia: mapping the literature by bibliometric analysis. Int J Geriatr Psychiatry 2003; 18: 41-54

Bayer AJ, Fish M. The doctor's duty to the elderly patient in clinical trials. Drugs Aging 2003; 20: 1087-97.

Berghmans RLP, Ter Meulen RHJT. Ethical issues in research with dementia patients. Int J Geriatr Psychiatry 1995; 10: 647-51.

Brooker D. What is person-centred care in dementia? Rev Clin Geront 2004;

Cassel CK, Jameton AL. Dementia in the elderly: an analysis of medical responsibility. Ann Intern Med 1981: 94; 802-807.

Downs M. The emergence of the person in dementia research. Aging and Society,1997; 17: 597-607

High DM, Whitehouse PJ, Post SG, Berg L. Guidelines for addressing ethical and legal issues in Alzheimer disease research: a position paper. Alz Dis Assoc Disord 1994; 8(S4): 66-74

Hughes JC. Views of the person with dementia. Journal of Medical Ethics, 2001:27; 86-91

Innes A. (editor) Dementia Care Mapping: Applications across cultures. Baltimore: Health Services Press, 2003

Kitwood T, Bredin, K. Towards a theory of Dementia care: Personhood and wellbeing. Ageing and Society,1992: **12**; 269-87

Kitwood T. Dementia Reconsidered: the person comes first. Buckingham: Open University Press, 1997.

Post S. The Moral Challenge of Alzheimer's disease. Baltimore: John Hopkins University Press, 1995

4.2

MEMORY CLINICS

Specialised out-patient clinics for older people with memory problems were first developed in the US and UK in the early 1980s. As well as offering a diagnostic, advice and treatment service, the clinics acted as a focus for education and research. The availability of specific drug treatment for AD has led to a rapid growth in their number and variety.

Why the need?

The development of a local Memory Clinic will have benefits for patients, their families, referring professionals, other local service providers and health and social service planners.

- In the past, services have tended to give a low priority to forgetful and people with mild dementia. This fails to recognise the potential of anticipatory, community-based care. By seeing people in the early stages of dementia, Memory Clinics enable informed decisions to be made about future care and need for intervention. Pre-emptive action before a crisis occurs will usually result in a better outcome and improved quality of life for all concerned.

- Forgetfulness is a common early sign of dementia, but often assumed to be merely due to ageing. Referral to a Memory Clinic, rather than a conventional psychiatric, neurological or geriatric service, is non-stigmatising and generally more acceptable to patients, families and referring professionals. The provision of a specialist service helps to raise local awareness, promoting improved lay and professional recognition and care of dementia.

Table *Benefits of Memory Clinics*

Benefits for patients and families

- Early identification and intervention
- Specialist assessment and robust diagnosis
- Anti-dementia drugs are effectively targeted, monitored and stopped when appropriate
- Education and support for patients and carers
- Anxiety management
- Advice on memory aids and memory training
- Access to research studies

Benefits for service providers

- Encourages earlier referral and develops awareness of dementia in primary care
- Standardised assessment and diagnosis
- Efficient targeting and monitoring of medication
- Facilitates audit and evaluation of services
- Addresses increasing demand for expert diagnosis and treatment
- Focus for research activity

- The assessment of mild cognitive impairment and the differential diagnosis of early dementia is not straightforward. A multi-disciplinary approach providing detailed, specialist assessment of referred cases is most successful. Robust diagnosis is assured and intervention can be effectively targeted.

- Earlier awareness of the needs and wants of people with dementia and of their families encourages better planning and provision of local health and social services. Postponement of institutionalisation by even a few months may have economic as well as psycho-social benefits.

- The availability of effective drug treatment for AD and some other forms of dementia demands a greater urgency for diagnosis at an early stage, when intervention is likely to be most beneficial.

- The UK National Service Framework for Older People (NSF) considers the inclusion of Memory Clinic services to be an essential component of hospital-based health services.

How do they work?

Characteristically, Memory Clinics are multi-disciplinary in nature, with patients and relatives being seen jointly by a physician and psychologist. Some clinics may also regularly involve nurses, speech therapists, occupational therapists or social workers.

- Memory Clinics should be held close to the community they serve. Holding them in easily accessible and acceptable sites, away from the more intimidating surroundings of specialist hospital centres, helps to encourage referral and attendance.

- Patients should be asked to come to the clinic with someone who knows them well and can provide a corroborative history.

- The procedure is then:

    - to take a full medical and social history from the patient and independently from the accompanying relative or friend.

    - to complete an appropriate physical examination, with particular attention to the cardiovascular, central nervous system and special senses

    - to confirm and quantify objective evidence of memory and other intellectual deficits. Testing usually starts with a brief general assessment of global mental function, such as the MMSE and then proceeds to more sensitive and specific brief measures of individual cognitive functions. This battery should ideally be completed on at least two occasions a few weeks apart. Much more detailed neuropsychological assessment may be appropriate in the minority of patients with atypical features. Particular attention needs to be given to excluding a mood disorder.

- To arrange appropriate laboratory, radiological and electrophysiological investigations. Structural neuroimaging should be an integral part of the assessment in most cases, whenever possible.

- By the second or third clinic visit, it should be possible to formulate a working diagnosis and this is then discussed with patient and family. Explanation and general counselling, supplemented by written information are given. Advice on management, any necessary referrals to other agencies and arrangement for community services can be made. Existing medication can be rationalised and new treatment introduced where indicated. Patients should then be offered future follow up according to local circumstances.

- A dedicated Community-based Memory Team (perhaps consisting of nurse, psychologist and social worker), working closely with the Memory Clinic Staff, will help to ensure patients and families get continuing help and support and timely involvement of other available services. This will help to reduce domestic stress and avoid unnecessary and premature institutionalisation.

FURTHER READING AND REFERENCES

Ames D, Flicker L, Helme RD. A memory clinic at a geriatric hospital: rationale, routine and results from the first 100 patients. Medical Journal of Australia 1992; 156: 618-622.

Bayer AJ, Richards V, Phillips G. The community memory project - a multidisciplinary approach to patients with forgetfulness and early dementia. Care of the Elderly 1990; 2(6):236-238.

Bayer AJ, Pathy MS, Twining C. The memory clinic. A new approach to the detection of early dementia. Drugs. 1987;33 Suppl 2:84-9.

Fraser, M. Memory clinics and memory training. In: Arie T (ed) Recent Advances in Psychogeriatrics, Edinburgh, Curchill Livingstone 1992, 105-115.

Hodges JR, Berrios GE, Breen K. The multidisciplinary memory clinic approach. In: Berrios GE, Hodges JR (eds). Memory Disorders in psychiatric practice. Cambridge, Cambridge University Press 2000. 101-21

Høgh P, Waldemar G, Knudsen GM et al. A multidisciplinary memory clinic in a neurological setting. Diagnostic evaluation of 400 consecutive patients. European Journal of Neurology 1999; 6: 279-288.

Lindesay J, Marundar M, et al. The second Leicester survey of memory clinics in the British Isles. Int J Geriatr Psychiatry 2002; 17: 41-7.

Logiudice D, Waltrowic W, Brown K, et al. Do memory clinics improve the quality of life of carers? A randomised controlled pilot study. Int J Geriatr Psychiatry 1999; 14: 626-32.

Philpot, M.P. and Levy, R. A memory clinic for the early diagnosis of dementia. Int. J.Geriatr.Psychiatry 1987; 2:195-200.

Twining TC. The Memory Handbook. Bicester: Winslow Press, 1993.

Van der Cammen, T.J.M., Simpson, J.M., Fraser, R.M., Preker, A.S. and Exton-Smith, A.N. The memory clinic: a new approach to the detection of dementia. Br.J.Psychiatry 1987; 150:359-364.

Voss SE, Bullock RA, Elcock J. A memory clinic in a department of old-age psychiatry: its role in clinical and academic research. International Journal of Psychiatry in Clinical Practice 1999; 3: 193197.

Wilcock GK, Bucks RS, Rockwood K.(eds.) Diagnosis and management of dementia. A manual for memory disorders teams. Oxford, Oxford University Press 1999.

Wright N, Lindesay J. A survey of memory clinics in the British isles. Int J Geriatr Psychiatry 1995; 10: 379-85.

4.3

MULTIDISCIPLINARY APPROACH TO CARE

During the course of a dementing illness, multiple medical, psychological and social needs will inevitably arise. Optimal care will therefore best be delivered by involvement of a variety of professionals, each able to contribute their different skills and expertise. By successfully working together, a multidisciplinary team can deliver a service that is greater than the sum of its parts.

Members Of The Multidisciplinary Team

Professionals involved in providing care to demented patients and their families will include:

- **Family doctor**, often best placed to co-ordinate involvement of other services and able to deal with day-to-day medical care. Initially the doctor should provide a working diagnosis that will help to focus management and guide prognosis. Medical crises should be foreseen and averted whenever possible.

- **Specialist geriatric, psychiatric or neurological opinions** can be sought, depending on local availability and ease of access. When possible, an initial specialist assessment to confirm diagnosis, exclude treatable causes of dementia and advise on management of specific problems is desirable. Medical management can then revert to the responsibility of the general practitioner, with specialist involvement if problematic behaviour develops.

- **Psychologists** can initially help with detailed neuropsychological assessment to identify deficits and aid the diagnostic process. Repeated assessment helps to monitor subsequent change. After diagnosis, psychologists may contribute to management of both patient and carers, including advice on mood disturbance and stress management, behavioural techniques and use of reality orientation, reminiscence and validation approaches.

- **Speech and language specialists, occupational therapists and physiotherapists** can offer invaluable help in their own specialist areas, particularly with prevention and maintenance activities. **Dieticians and dentists** will play an important role when nutrition and dental care have been neglected.

- **Community-based nursing and home care services** can provide help with day to day practical management, for example helping with personal care, bathing, administering medication, changing dressings and advice and support to carers. There is a need for such services to be flexible and able to respond rapidly to changing and unforeseen needs. In some areas, **specialist community psychiatric nurses** may be available to provide advice on management of persistent, difficult behaviours.

- **Social workers** can advise carers on the choices available, ensure all financial assistance is forthcoming and ensure that involvement of community and residential care services is both timely and appropriate. Helping relatives to understand and come to terms with the implications of dementia may be very time consuming. A proactive rather than reactive approach is most successful, negotiating, co-ordinating and monitoring an acceptable package of care services.

- **Alzheimer's Disease Society** groups can provide invaluable advice and support. Other **voluntary and church organisations** may provide sitting services, help with transport, organisation of carer's support groups, social outings or supply of mobility and toileting aids. **Local priests** may sometimes be key movers in mobilising and gaining acceptance for service involvement. The **private sector** may be able to provide (at a cost) an individualised home care and support service.

Multidisciplinary Methods Of Working

Features of successful multidisciplinary working include:

- **good communications** between all team members and with other agencies involved in delivering care. Individual responsibilities need to be clear, ensuring a collaborative approach to delivery of optimum care. Formal liaison between agencies and agreement over service demarcation will help to minimise disputes. There is a need for regular team meetings to discuss individual and general approaches to care.

- **a named key worker** to co-ordinate care. Poorly organised service involvement, duplication of effort and inter-professional rivalry can then be avoided, with good case management leading to development of individualised care packages.

- **a team leader** able to foster mutual respect and trust between members, to maximise individual strengths and to create compromise when appropriate. The motivation of the team as a whole will often depend on the strength of leadership.

- **realistic goals**, based on available resources. This helps to give a practical framework and sense of purpose to delivery of care.

- **mutual respect and trust** between team members, providing support and encouragement for each other. All should accept that they are each dependent on the expertise of others and no single professional has all the answers. Highlighting individual strengths as much as weaknesses will help to maintain morale.

- **constant evolution**, with regular self-assessment identifying good and bad practices and opportunity and encouragement to incorporate new ideas. Meeting training needs and continuing education of all team members is crucial.

FURTHER READING AND REFERENCES

Audit Commission. Forget me Not. Mental Health Services for Older People. London, Audit Commission 2000.

Bartels SJ, Dums AR, Oxman TE, et al. Evidence-based practices in geriatric mental health care.Psychiatr Serv. 2002;53:1419-31.

Beck CK, Cody M, Zhang M. A multidisciplinary team approach to managing Alzheimer's disease. Pharmacotherapy. 1998;18(2 Pt 2):33-42; discussion 79-82.

Challis D, Reilly S, Hughes J, et al. Policy, organisation and practice of specialist old age psychiatry in England. Int J Geriatr Psychiatry. 2002;17:1018-26

Grossberg GT, Lake JT. The role of the psychiatrist in Alzheimer's disease. J Clin Psychiatry. 1998;59 Suppl 9:3-6.

Jurkowski CL.A multidisciplinary approach to Alzheimer's disease: who should be members of the team? Am J Med. 1998;104(4A): 13S-16S; discussion 39S-42S.

Lloyd-Williams M, Payne S. Can multidisciplinary guidelines improve the palliation of symptoms in the terminal phase of dementia? Int J Palliat Nurs. 2002;8:370-5.

4.4

DIAGNOSTIC DISCLOSURE AND MEETING INFORMATION NEEDS

The culture of dementia diagnosis and disclosure is changing, with increased public awareness of dementia (many patients and families consider the possibility prior to diagnosis), earlier referral and diagnosis, increasing accuracy of modern diagnostic criteria (now approaching 90% in specialist centres) and the availability of effective symptomatic treatment.

Telling the Diagnosis

- Most advocates for people with dementia and their carers now believe that, in most cases, patients should be told what is wrong with them, what the implications are, what can be done for them and what treatment is likely to involve.
- Carers also need good quality advice and information, provided at the right time and in suitable formats and languages, as well as easy access to support services.
- An early and accurate diagnosis of dementia is vital for patients and carers. The right of all patients to have access to comprehensive assessment and to know the outcome is now a well established priority. At the same time, patients are individuals and have a right also not to know if that is their wish.

- All must be given the opportunity to learn as much or as little as they want to know. It is not for professionals to decide, but to provide information and support.

Attitudes To Diagnosis Disclosure

- There is no consistency in current clinical practice concerning telling patients with dementia of their diagnosis. Increasingly in Northern European countries it is becoming the accepted standard of care, whereas in Southern and Eastern Europe it is still the exception rather than the rule. A recent survey of carers of people with AD or other dementia in 11 European countries found that in 46% of cases, diagnosis had been disclosed to the family only and not to the patient, 46% of carers found information provided to them was insufficient and 29% subsequently had no regular contact with any health professional.

- Practice of diagnosis disclosure amongst dementia specialists is changing. Ten years ago, 32% of old age psychiatrists and 24% of geriatricians "usually told" people with mild dementia their diagnosis, though 12% or less told those with moderate or severe dementia. More recent studies report that 40-50% of specialists now regularly disclose diagnosis, whilst 20% see no benefit in doing so.

- A recent study in general practice conducted in the U.K. reported that 39% of GPs always or often informed patients about a diagnosis of dementia (whereas 95% would now inform a patient with terminal cancer, compared with only 2% 30 years ago). About the same proportion would discuss prognosis.

- Family members' attitudes toward telling patients with AD their diagnosis are inconsistent, with most not wanting the patient to be told (because of fears that the knowledge would depress or agitate them, that they would not understand, or that there was no benefit in knowing), whereas most would themselves want to be told if they developed AD (considering that it was their right to know and that it would enable them to plan for the future). The difference may arise because of a reluctance of relatives to deal with patients' knowledge and possible grief, a paternalistic desire to protect the patient from reality, or perhaps a generational difference in perception of AD.

- Reactions of AD patients to being told their diagnosis include relief (as the diagnosis provides an explanation for their difficulties), disbelief (as they may lack insight and do not feel ill), loss (grieving for failing intellectual abilities and limitations in the future) and fear of becoming a burden.

Table *Arguments for and against disclosure of a diagnosis of dementia*

AGAINST DISCLOSURE

- making an accurate diagnosis is complex and uncertain in the absence of neuropathology
- there is no curative intervention
- giving such a diagnosis causes avoidable anxiety and depression
- people with AD will not be able to remember and use the information given to them.

FOR DISCLOSURE

- maximizes individual autonomy and choice by providing information necessary for decision making and advance planning
- increases opportunities for accessing appropriate and specialist support services and symptomatic treatments
- demonstrates respect for individual rights, especially the 'right to know' and avoids paternalism
- relieves the anxiety of uncertainty

- The circumstances when it may be inappropriate to talk about diagnosis include:
    - when dementia is severe and understanding of the diagnosis is unlikely
    - when a phobia about the condition is likely
    - when a patient is severely depressed
    - when patients clearly state they do not wish to know

Telling The Diagnosis

The following recommendations may be made:

- Communication of the diagnosis should ordinarily occur in a **joint meeting with patient and family**
- Use **simple language**. Avoid technical jargon that may conceal the truth.
- **Use a graded approach** which is patient led and allows the information given to be matched to what the patient wants to know.
- **Allow sufficient time** to explain and to answer questions from the patient and family.
- Assess the patient's and the family's **understanding**_and arrange **follow up** (to reinforce information provided, clarify misunderstandings and answer questions that are outstanding)
- **Use the term "Alzheimer's disease"** (or other appropriate medical diagnosis) rather than just dementia and ensure that they understand the sense of both terms
- **Mellow the bad news** with the possibility of therapeutic approaches (not just drugs). Avoid conveying the feeling that "nothing more can be done"

- Make it clear that a reorganised family network can **alleviate burden and maintain quality of life**.

- **Inform the patient** about the possibility to take decisions about his/her future

Information Provision

- As well as clearly describing diagnosis, specific attention should be given to comprehensible and practical information about coping strategies, care services, likely course of the disease and treatment, specific drug treatment and follow up

- Most people much prefer to receive information face-to-face from an informed professional. This is not only a medical responsibility. All members of the multi-disciplinary team should consider every therapeutic encounter to be an opportunity for education and information provision.

- Dedicated time should be put aside during the consultation for information provision – it should never be merely an after-thought at the end of the assessment.

- Verbal information should be backed up by written information, with recommendations for further reading. Increasingly people are turning to the internet for more detailed information and trustworthy websites should be recommended to those interested. Mention should be made of local support groups and meetings and contact details of local Alzheimer support organisations.

- Patients and carers both have individual needs and each should be addressed separately.

FURTHER READING AND REFERENCES

Audit Commission. Forget-me-not: mental health services for older people. London, Audit Commission, 2000.

Harris M, Bayer A, Tadd W. Addressing the information needs of older patients. Rev Clin Geront 2002; 12:

Drickamer MA, Lachs MS. Should patients with Alzheimer's disease be told their diagnosis? NEJM 1992: 326: 947-51.

Fearnley K, McLennan J, Weaks D. The Right to Know? Sharing the diagnosis of dementia. Edinburgh: Alzheimer Scotland – Action on Dementia 1997.

Gilliard J and Gwilliam C. Sharing the diagnosis: a survey of memory disorder clinics, their policies on informing people with dementia dn their families, and the support they offer. Int J Geriatr Psychiatry 1996; 11: 1001-1003.

Holroyd S, Snustad DG and Chalifoux ZL. Attitudes of older adults' on being told the diagnosis of AD. J Am Geriatr Soc 1996; 44: 440-403.

Marzanski, M. Would you like to know what is wrong with your? On telling the truth to patients with dementia. J Med Ethics. 2000; 26; 108-113.

Maguire CP, Kirby M, Coen R, Coakley D, Lawlor BA, O'Neill D. Family members' attitudes toward telling the patient with Alzheimer's disease their diagnosis. BMJ 1996; 313: 529-30.

OPDAL Study Group. Optimisation of the Diagnosis of Alzheimer's Disease Luxembourg, Alzheimer Europe 2003

Pratt R, Wilkinson H. 'Tell me the truth'. The effect of being told the diagnosis of dementia from the perspective of the person with dementia. London, Mental Health Foundation 2001.

Rice K and Warner N. Breaking the bad news: what do psychiatrists tell patients with dementia about their illness? Int J Geri Psychiatry: 1994; 9: 467-471.

Woods RT, Moniz-Cook E, Iliffe S, et al. Dementia: issues in early recognition and intervention in primary care. J Royal Society Med 2003; 96: 320-4.

4.5

DRUG TREATMENT

General Considerations

As the aetiology of dementing illnesses is so varied, no one drug is likely to be beneficial in all patients. The choice of medication should clearly relate to the underlying condition or the specific symptom that is to be treated.

- Many drugs may positively influence some symptoms, but have an adverse effect on others (e.g. neuroleptics may help agitation, but worsen cognition). Careful initial assessment and investigation is therefore essential before any pharmacological intervention is considered. Subsequently, the impact of treatment and the indication for its continuing use must be kept under regular review.

- The size of any drug effect that can be considered worthwhile is open to debate. A slight improvement in memory may be very valuable in patients early in the course of the illness, but of little impact when other symptoms have come to dominate the clinical picture. Statistically significant improvement on psychometric tests does not necessarily equate with meaningful change in quality of life. A noticeable improvement or stabilisation is more important than change in test score.

- Patients and carers tend to be more positive than professionals when assessing apparently small benefits of treatment, with three quarters believing that halting progression of symptoms of early dementia for about six months would tend to justify intervention. Such modest effect would seem comparable to that achieved by the drugs now available to treat AD.

- A minority of dementing conditions can be effectively halted or reversed by specific drug treatment. For example, hypothyrodism by thyroxine, pernicious anaemia by parenteral vitamin B12, neurosyphilis by penicillin, cerebral vasculitis by cortiocosteroids or immunosuppressants and Wernicke-Korsakoff's syndrome and possibly alcoholic dementia by thiamine. However, truly reversible dementia is probably rare.

- In AD and VaD, the risk of vascular events can be reduced by judicious use of anti-hypertensive medication, treatment of hyperlipidaemia and anti-platelet drugs (e.g. low dose aspirin). Oral anticoagulation should be considered in patients with a source of emboli, such as valvular heart disease or atrial fibrillation and in whom the risk of bleeding events is thought to be acceptable.

- In DLB and PDD, dopaminergic drug therapy does not improve cognition and can even worsen confusion. Particular care is needed with use of neuroleptic drugs in these patients, who are especially sensitive to their effects.

Drug treatment of non-cognitive symptoms

The non-cognitive, neuropsychiatric symptoms of dementia can be especially troublesome to carers and, when used judiciously, drugs can reduce patients' and families' distress and delay or prevent the need for institutionalisation.

- The acetylcholinesterase inhibitor drugs can favourably influence a range of neuropsychiatric symptoms and should generally be considered as first choice in non-urgent situations.

- Neuroleptic drugs are commonly used and are modestly effective in treating agitation, aggression, delusions and hallucinations. However, there is little evidence from clinical trials to suggest the optimum dose, duration of treatment, or differential efficacy of the various agents available. Side effects can be problematic, including sedation, anticholinergic toxicity, postural hypertension, Parkinsonism, akathisia and dyskinesias. They tend to be dose related and are especially common with depot preparations, when combined with other drug treatments and in DLB. The atypical drugs (risperidone, olanzapine, quetiepine) have become the neuroleptic drugs of first choice, due to their lower incidence of extrapyramidal effects. Starting doses should be very low (e.g. risperidone 0.5mg or haloperidol 0.5mg) and titrated against the clinical state.

- Non-neuroleptic drugs to treat behavioural disturbance have seldom been assessed in clinical trials, but there is anecdotal evidence of efficacy in some patients. Their role in routine management is uncertain. Drugs used have included lithium, carbamazepine, benzodiazepines trazodone, and beta-blockers (propranolol, pindolol).

- Sleep disturbance may justify use of a short acting hypnotic such as zopiclone, or a small dose of trazodone.

- Depressive symptoms should be actively treated and about three quarters of depressed, demented patients will respond to appropriate antidepressant drugs. The newer SSRIs are the antidepressants of first choice. Trazodone is a useful alternative in the anxious patient with sleep disturbance.

Acetylcholinesterase inhibitors (AChEI)

Acetylcholinesterase inhibitor (AChEI) drugs that inhibit the breakdown of acetylcholine within the synapse, increasing its availability to muscarinic and nicotinic receptors, have become the mainstay of treatment for AD, and may also have benefits in DLB, PDD and VaD.

- Early AChEI drugs, such as physostigmine, were shown to have limited efficacy in AD, but were poorly tolerated.

tacrine was the first AChEI to be licensed specifically for AD, but is poorly tolerated with 30-40% patients having a specific but reversible hepatotoxicity and also a high incidence of dose-related cholinergic side effects. It has been superseded by the newer agents, donepezil (Aricept), rivastigmine (Exelon) and galantamine (Reminyl).

- **Donepezil** is highly selective for AChE with a long plasma half-life allowing once daily dosing. Patients commence on 5mg per day which can be increased to 10mg after at least 4 weeks to reduce the risk of side-effects.

- **Rivastigmine** inactivates AChE and butyrylcholinesterase (BuChE) for about 10 hours, so can be given twice daily despite a short plasma half-life. It appears to be especially active in the cortex and hippocampus and preferentially inhibits the G1 form of AChE that is relatively more abundant in the brain in AD. Inhibition of BuChE as well as AchE offers theoretical advantages, though clinical benefit has yet to be proven. It is given with food beginning at 1.5mg bd and increasing gradually to the effective dose range of 3-6 mg bd.

- **Galantamine** is more active against AChE than BuChE but less so than donepezil. It is given twice daily, preferably with food, starting with a non-therapeutic dose of 4mg bd for 4 weeks before increasing to therapeutic dose levels of 16-24mg per day. Galantamine has also been shown to modulate nicotinic receptors and it has been suggested this may provide additional clinical efficacy.

- In AD, donepezil, rivastigmine and galantamine have all been shown to be statistically better than treatment with placebo, with improvements in cognition, ADL and and overall clinical global impression and with positive effect on aspects of behaviour such as apathy, anxiety, hallucinations and agitation. There is also evidence of efficacy in more severe AD and suggestion of potential savings in healthcare costs, carer time and burden and delay in need for permanent institutional care. Clinical trials have also been conducted in patients with mixed dementia, VaD, DLB and PDD. Preliminary results suggest that they are efficacious and safe in these conditions.

- All AChEIs have qualitatively similar cholinergic adverse effects, including nausea, vomiting, diarrhoea, fatigue and dizziness. These are generally mild and short-lived, resolving despite continued therapy. Caution with use of AChEIs should be observed in the presence of bradycardia and atrial or ventricular conduction disorders. Muscle cramps, insomnia and nightmares are more common with donepezil and can sometimes be reduced by administering the drug in the morning rather than at night.

- About 40-60% of AD patients respond to AchEIs. So far similarities appear to be greater than the differences between the available AChEIs, but it may be reasonable to consider switching drugs if patients do not tolerate or respond to the first drug used.

Table *Pharmacotherapy of Alzheimer's disease (2004)*

Proven efficacy
- Cholinesterase inhibitors (donepezil, rivastigmine, galantamine)
- Memantine

Uncertain efficacy
- Vitamin E, Selegiline, Ginkgo biloba, Statins, Anti-inflammatory drugs, Neurotrophins, Secretase inhibitors, Immunotherapy, Stem cells therapy

No efficacy (or doubtful)
- Vasodilators
- Lecitihin/choline
- Nootropics
- Cholinergic agonists
- Steroids
- Oestrogen

Memantine

Glutaminergic overstimulation and consequent calcium overload has been implicated in neurodegeneration.

- Memantine is a non-competitive NMDA (glutamate) receptor antagonist that blocks pathologically elevated glutamate, so offering neuroprotection, whilst still allowing physiological receptor activation. The drug has recently become available for treatment of moderately severe to severe AD and there is also preliminary evidence of efficacy in milder AD and VaD.

- In clinical trials in patients with severe AD, patients taking memantine showed significantly less deterioration in functional, cognitive and global measures and need for institutionalization and demands on caregiver time were significantly reduced. The addition of memantine to donepezil treatment appears to show benefit over donepezil alone. Patients start on a once daily dose of 5mg, increasing gradually to the effective dose range of 10 mg bd. Memantine appears to be safe and very well tolerated, despite the advanced age and frailty of many of the treated patients.

Antioxidants

Antioxidants are thought to reduce free radical production and the excessive lipid peroxidation that can lead to neuronal damage. This is thought to be the likely mechanism supporting the use of vitamin E, selegiline and Ginkgo biloba.

- **Vitamin E**. In moderately severe AD, treatment with vitamin E delayed progression of the disease to significant endpoints (death, institutionalisation, loss of two out of three basic ADLs, or severe dementia) by 215-230 days., though number of reported falls was increased. This trial used very high doses (1000 IU twice daily) that may be associated with adverse effects. More conventional doses (200-800 IU per day) are generally recommended, although data for this are lacking.

- **Selegiline**. As well as its antoxidant activity, selegiline is a monoamine oxidase B inhibitor. A Cochrane review of its use in AD reported improvement in cognition, behaviour and mood, but little evidence of global or functional benefit. Selegiline is less well tolerated than vitamin E and care must be taken with concurrent tricyclic and SSRI antidepressants. Use in AD is not generally recommended.

- **Gingko biloba**. Extracts from the leaves of the gingko biloba tree have been used in China for thousands of years, but as the extracts contain a range of ingredients it is difficult to identify the active substance or which action is important. Gingko extracts are popular in Europe but most clinical trials have been of poor quality and there is limited evidence of efficacy. Mild gastrointestinal complaints, headache and allergic skin reactions are uncommon and there have been rare reports of bleeding complications. Numerous gingko preparations are available and their composition may vary. Most trials have used an extract called EGb761. The usual dose range is 120-240mg.

Anti-inflammatory agents

Inflammatory mechanisms are important in AD and possibly in atherosclerotic conditions. Acute-phase proteins and complement are associated with amyloid deposits and activated microglial cells may be important in the conversion of diffuse plaques to neuritic plaques in AD. One meta-analysis of epidemiological studies suggested that anti-inflammatory treatment might decrease the risk of developing AD by as much as 50%. Whilst a small trial of indometacin appeared to confirm potential efficacy in AD, larger trials of NSAIDs, COX-2 inhibitors, prednisone and hydroxychloroquine have all been negative. Newer anti-inflammatory agents are under investigation.

Oestrogen Replacement Therapy

Depite epidemiological studies strongly suggesting that hormone replacement therapy in post-menopausal women improved cognitive function, delayed the onset of dementia and reduced severity of cognitive decline, this has not been confirmed in any prospective randomized placebo controlled trial. Indeed, the large prospective Women's Health Study showed an increased risk of stroke and dementia associated with use of combined HRT. Thus its use for treatment or prevention of dementia is not supported by current evidence.

Statins

Recent epidemiological reports have described an association between therapy with statins and a reduction in the occurrence of AD by as much as 70%. This is supported by a growing body of biological and clinical evidence that lowering serum cholesterol may retard the pathogenesis of AD. Prospective randomised placebo controlled trials are underway.

Folate, Vitamin B12 and homocysteine

An elevated serum total homocysteine level is a risk factor for vascular disease and probably for AD. High homocysteine levels are associated with low folate and vitamin B12 levels. No prospective randomised controlled trials of folic acid and/or vitamin B12 supplements have been completed.

Potential new treatments

Immunotherapy. Antibodies to beta amyloid increase its clearance from the brain. In transgenic mice models of AD. Prophylactic immunization, even by nasal applicayion of an amyloid fragment, reduces plaque formation and protects against learning and memory impairments. Initial clinical trials in AD patients confirmed that an antibody response to beta amyloid could be generated and preliminary results suggest a reduction in plaque formation similar to that seen in animal experiments and possibly some slowing of functional decline. However, trials were discontinued because of a 5-8% incidence of encephalitis in treatment subjects, probably mediated by a T-cell response. Modifications of the vaccine are being made and further studies will follow.

Secretase inhibitors. Beta and gamma secretase are critical enzymes in the production of beta amyloid. Mice that lack beta secretase do not produce beta amyloid but develop normally, suggesting that beta secretase inhibition has therapeutic potential in AD. Several small molecule inhibitors of beta secretase capable of crossing the blood brain barrier are under development. Gamma secretase inhibitors can selectively inhibit APP breakdown and decrease amyloid production and presenilin gene mutations result in altered gamma secretase and early onset AD. However, mice that lack gamma secretase die in utero, raising caution about its value as a therapeutic target.

Neurotrophic Agents (nerve growth factor, NGF) In animals, NGF promotes survival of cholinergic cells, reverses atrophy and improves memory in models of Alzheimer's disease. Recently NGF receptors have been demonstrated in human brain and biotechnology is producing a more dependable source of NGF. However, there is no easy method of drug delivery (an intraventricular pump would probably be required). Furthermore there is a suggestion that high neurotrophic activity may occur in response to degenerative change, itself contributing to the pathogenesis of Alzheimer's disease.

Stem cell therapy. Most neurones in the adult CNS are terminally differentiated and are not replaced by new neurones when they die. Neural stem cells, however, persist in the adult brain subventricular zone and continually generate large number of neurones and glial cells. Small populations of neurones are also formed in the adult olfactory bulb and hippocampus. Newly born neurones originate from putative stem cells that exist in the subgranular zone of the dentate gyrus. This late neurogenesis continues throughout adult life, but decreases with stress and during aging. An enriched environment, mental activity, physical activity and even antidepressants increase neurogenesis. Further research into the regulation of stem cell proliferation and differentiation will allow the development of new strategies to stimulate neurogenesis in the adult brain.

Stem cells can also be harvested from a variety of brain and spinal cord regions and transplanted back into the brain or spinal cord where these cells can differentiate into mature glia or neurones depending on the local environment. Cells can be harvested from adult brains, fetal brains or from the inner cell mass of in vitro fertilized blastocysts and can be differentiated in vitro using various growth factors to affect their differentiation. There is now evidence that umbilical cord blood and bone marrow cells are pluripotent progenitor cells, which can be driven to differentiate into cell lineages that are not part of their hematopoetic repertoire. Both cell sources have a relatively high commitment to differentiate into neural tissues. Therefore, rebuilding functional tissue in CNS diseases could be achieved through the directed homing of umbilical blood or bone marrow progenitor cells into diseased brain or spinal cord. Clinical trials are underway to investigate the potential for treatment of ischemic brain lesions and spinal cord injury.

Neurotransplantation. Current research focuses on potential of neural grafts to replace damaged or missing cell populations, on delivery of growth factors and on delivery of needed gene products through transgenes. Cell replacement therapy for PD assumes that implanted dopaminergic neurones may substitute for the loss of nigrostriatal neurons. Clinical trials have shown that dopamine neuroblasts obtained from fetal human mesencephalon can survive and function in the brain of PD patients, restore striatal dopamine release and ameliorate impairments in motor behaviour. However, progenitor cells taken at earlier stages of development might prove more effective and can be expanded in vitro. Thus a variety of neurodegenerative diseases might be treated with cell replacement therapy, but each may require different neurtransplantation strategies.

Tissue engineering. Combining cell transplantation with bioengineering techniques may offer new sources of cells for replacement therapy. Besides the direct implantation of cells to diseased regions and their injections into the CSF or intravenously, neural stem cells can be cultured in vitro on biocompatible carriers and then enter and populate in the CNS parenchyma in a multifocal fashion. When combined with synthetic biomaterials and growth factors, neural stem cells can be even more effective in engineering the damaged CNS towards reconstitution.

FURTHER READING AND REFERENCES

Bullock R. New drugs for Alzheimer's disease and other dementias. Br J Psychiatry 2002; 180: 135-9.

Jones RW. Drug Treatment of Dementia. Oxford: Blackwell Science, 2000

Le Bars PL, Katz MM, Berman N et al. A placebo-controlled, double-blind, randomised trial of an extract of Ginkgo biloba for dementia. JAMA 1997; 278: 1327-32.

Livingston G, Katona C. How useful are cholinesterase inhibitors in the treatment of Alzheimer's disease? A number needed to treat analysis. Int J Geriat Psychiatry 2000;15: 203-7.

McGeer PL, McGeer EG. The inflammatory response system of brain: implications for therapy of Alzheimer's and other neurodegenerative diseases. Brain Res Rev 1995; 21: 195-218

National Institute for Clinical Excellence. Guidance on the use of Donepezil, Rivastigmine and Galantamine for the Treatment of Alzheimer's disease. London: NICE, 2001

Sano M, Ernesto C, Thomas RG et al. A controlled trial of selegiline, alpha-tocopherol, or both as treatment for Alzheimer's disease. N Eng J Med 1997; 336: 1216-22.

Scott HD, Laake K. Statins for the prevention of Alzheimer's disease (Cochrane Review). In: The Cochrane Library, 1, 2002. Oxford: Update Software.

Schneider LS. Treatment of Alzheimer's Disease with Cholinesterase Inhibitors. Clinics Geriatr Med 2001; 17: 337-58.

Zigova T., Snyder E. Y., Sanberg P.R.(Editors) Neural Stem Cells for Brain and Spinal Cord Repair. Totowa, New Jersey, Humana Press, pp. 1-434, 2003.

4.6

COGNITIVE TRAINING

The idea of cognitive training as a method of improving, retaining or regaining skills is attractive to those worried about memory loss and to relatives who hope that developing problems might be minimised. Recent evidence suggesting that education and continued intellectual activity may reduce the risk of developing Alzheimer's disease has further increased interest in this area.

Experience of formal training programmes designed to improve the cognitive skills of healthy elderly subjects and those with dementia is limited. Those most likely to gain appear to be well-motivated, healthy individuals wishing to conserve their mental faculties as a prophylactic measure. There is little evidence of sustained benefit or generalisability in those with established dementia and regular tests and 'exercises' for the memory can easily become counterproductive. Positive benefits to patients may even be at the cost of increased distress to carers.

Specific approaches to memory training have included:

- relaxation techniques
- regular and repeated practice sessions, using spaced retrieval to rehearse information
- organisation of material (e.g. use of categorisation, or mnemonics)
- techniques for improving visual imagery (e.g. pegword methods, face-name association etc.)

- verbal strategies (rhymes, first letter cueing, alphabet searching etc.)

- computer-aided cognitive training (sometimes combined with pharmacological treatment)

Training in groups with other people with memory impairment or with family members and carers may provide opportunities to harness a wider range of training resources and facilitate expression of mutual support. Another approach is to involve family members in providing the cognitive training at home.

The most simple and effective methods of helping patients (other than asking other people to remember things for them) are:

- **establishment of everyday routines**. This may mean keeping to a regular time-table through the day and week. If a routine is established, it is easier to mentally retrace a sequence of events when something is overlooked.

- **careful organisation of daily activities**. Learning to always put things away carefully in their own place is helpful. Out of date newspapers and other clutter should be thrown away. In the kitchen, use of a microwave cooker may avoid food being burnt in a conventional oven. Wall charts and display boards can reinforce the planned sequence of activity.

- **use of environmental cues**. Labelling or colour coding of switches and doors may sometimes be useful. Red warning lights on electrical appliances may help to remind when they are on, and use of kettles that whistle may ensure that open pans do not boil dry. A timer or digital alarm watch may act as a reminder to take medication, or attend to cooking or other household tasks, or to refer to an appointments diary for guidance as to planned activities.

- **use of external memory aids**. Systematic use of written aids such as diaries, checklists and carefully positioned notes as reminders are often of benefit. Reusable sticky note pads are ideal for sticking in conspicuous places. Electronic devices and programmable organisers are generally too complicated and unfamiliar to prove useful.

None of these approaches require the patient to learn new strategies of thinking or remembering and may thus be potentially useful in those with mild dementia.

FURTHER READING AND REFERENCES

Camp CJ, McKitrick LA. Memory interventions in Alzheimer's type dementia populations: methodological and theoretical issues. In: West RL, Sinnott JD (eds.) Everyday memory and ageing New York: Springer-Verlag, 1993.

Clare L, Wilson BA, Carter G, et al. Intervening with everyday memory problems in early Alzheimer's disease: an errorless learning approach. J Clin Exp Neuropsychol 2000; 22: 132-146.

Clare L, Woods B, Moniz-Cook E, et al. Cognitive Rehabilitation interventions targeting memory functioning in early-stage Alzheimer's disease and vascular dementia. Cochrane Library, 2003.

Davis RN, Massman PJ, Doody RS. Cognitive intervention in Alzheimer Disease: a randomized placebo-controlled study. Alz Dis Assoc Disord 2001; 15: 1-9.

De Vreese LP, Neri M, Fioravanti M, et al. Memory rehabilitation in Alzheimer's disease: a review of progress. Int J Geriatr Psychiatry 2001; 16: 794-809.

Hill RD, Backman L, Neely AS (eds.) Cognitive Rehabilitation in Old Age Oxford, Oxford University Press, 2000.

Moore S, Sandman CA, McGrady K, et al. Memory training improves cognitive ability in patients with dementia. Neuropsychological Rehab 2001; 11: 245-61.

Quayhagen MP, Quayhagen M, Corbeil RR, et al. Coping with dementia: evaluation of four nonpharmacologic interventions. Int Psychogeriatrics 2000; 12: 249-65.

Wilson BA, Moffat N. Clinical Management of Memory Problems. London, Chapman and Hall, 1984.

4.7

MEMORY ALBUMS

A Memory Album is a visual record of the key facts of a person's life both past and present. Simple, clearly written sentences accompanied by photographs, postcards, newspaper cuttings, certificates etc. document the person's life chronologically.

A 'pocket-sized' photo album with about 36 plastic wallets can be made into a useful Memory Album. This is easy to carry around and is acceptable to people with dementia as it resembles more traditional memory aids such as diaries and notebooks. For patients with more advanced dementia, a larger album allows the use of larger photographs and captions which are more easily recognised

Putting a Memory Album together

- Ask the person with dementia and family members to gather together photographs, postcards, certificates etc. of the important people, places and events in the person's past and present life. Lay the material out chronologically

- Captions should then be devised which describe the material comprehensively but with few words. For example, the caption to a photograph might read 'MY SON JOHN. LONDON. 1978'. This reminds the person that he has a son, that his son is called John, that John was still a child in 1978 etc. An additional benefit of providing such detailed information is that it avoids embarrassment when someone looking through the album asks who John is and the patient is unable to answer.

- The captions should use adult language. A useful guideline is to ask yourself whether it would be acceptable to you.

- If someone has difficulty recognising a family member, a chronological series concerning that person could be included in the album. For example the following captions could accompany appropriate photographs:

(photograph)	(photograph)	(photograph)
MY HUSBAND BILL ON OUR WEDDING DAY 1957. BILL WAS 22.	BILL AND ME AT OUR SILVER WEDDING	BILL'S 40TH BIRTHDAY 1975

- Similarly, if someone continually says that his home is not really where he lives, the following series could be included in the album.

(photograph)	(photograph)
OUR OLD HOME IN FRANCE. WE LIVED HERE FOR 32 YEARS	28 RIVER ROW DUBLIN. WE MOVED HERE 5 YEARS AGO IN 1998

- New photographs and captions can be added to the album as significant life events occur. For people who move to residential care, it could be useful to include photographs (with appropriate captions) of the outside and inside of the building, along with photographs of staff and significant fellow residents, for example room-mates.

Potential Benefits of Using a Memory Album

- Keeps 'key facts' fresh - helping to preserve them in memory for as long as possible.

- Helps maintain sense of identity - offers a sense of security of knowing oneself. Builds self-esteem and confidence and makes the person feel his life is of value.

- Provides a focus for conversation and allows the person to take the lead. For early stage patients, it provides a method of self-prompting during conversation.

- Provides opportunity for life review and allows patient and carers to focus on the good times.

- Offers sense of security when the person moves on to day care or permanent care and helps staff to see the person as an individual, encouraging a more personalised approach to care. It also provides ideas for stimulating conversation.

Problems With Using a Memory Album

- Acceptance of the concept of a memory album can be a problem for some early stage patients and carers. Some carers are not able to cope with the logical thinking and organisation required to construct a well-ordered autobiography.

- Some carers and staff have difficulty understanding the purpose of a memory album and therefore may not encourage its use. Visual and perceptual problems may affect patient's ability to make sense of photos and captions. Even so, the album still provides useful information for staff.

FURTHER READING AND REFERENCES

Bourgeois MS. Conversing with memory impaired individuals using memory aids - a memory aid workbook. Bicester: Winslow Press, 1992

4.8

THERAPEUTIC APPROACHES

Psychological and complementary therapeutic approaches to management must recognise the individual differences between people with dementia patients and be carefully targeted to meet specific needs. No one approach will be suitable for all patients, or continue to suit any single patient throughout the course of their illness.

To be successful, treatment should be matched to patients' strengths as well as weaknesses and be able to flexibly adapt to the changing clinical situation. Ideally, the approach used should not require a lot of specialist professional input, but rather become an integral part of day to day activity and care.

- **Reminiscence** involves recall of events in a person's life, in conversation with another, in a group, or alone. Relevant pictures, music, objects and sounds are used to trigger the store of memories. It is certainly an enjoyable diversionary activity for patients and encourages staff to get to know more about patients as individuals. Proponents have reported benefits to include an increase in interaction, improved orientation and a reduction in behavioural disturbance. Reminiscence sessions can also be used to encourage patients to make a memory album.

- **Reality Orientation (RO)** provides information about the time, place or person to give the person with dementia a greater understanding of their situation, with the aim of improving sense of control and self-esteem. It often takes the form of structured group meetings, aiming to engage patients both with their immediate surroundings and with the world outside. An alternative approach is to provide 24 hour RO, by providing clocks, clear signposting, large notice boards and consistent information in all interactions with carers. Sustained improvement in verbal and spatial orientation has been claimed.

- **Validation therapy** emphasises the importance of relating to the inner reality of the patient, rather than encouraging them to be concerned with external factors. The therapist acknowledges and empathises with the patient's feelings, whether or not they are based on reality. The emphasis is on accepting and validating feelings rather than factual content. Validation can be delivered individually in formal sessions, as group therapy, or as 24 hour informal therapy. Evidence of efficacy is lacking and the underlying theoretical framework has been questioned.

- **Pet therapy** involves introducing pets, such as resident cats or visits by a dog, to institutionalised patients (provided that people are not scared by them). It can significantly increase the number of interactions whilst the therapy dog is present, producing longer conversations and increased rates of touch, as well as promoting a homely environment and facilitating the expression of emotions. Installation of fish tanks in the dining area of specialized dementia units has even been reported to increase nutritional intake and weight gain.

- **Music therapy** can be undertaken either individually using recorded tapes or simple instruments, or in groups using old songs or dance music. People respond best when th ey listen to music they prefer. Group music therapy can significantly improve speech content and fluency and some severely impaired patients may respond to music, even when other forms of communication have been lost. Several studies have showed that individualized music therapy can significantly decrease most forms of agitation. A recent study reported people with mild dementia had significantly improved scores on a visuo-spatial task after listening to 10 minutes of a Mozart piano sonata.

- **Physical exercise** may be undertaken either through informal walks or using structured exercise sessions. A study of walking combined with conversation in nursing home residents with dementia suggested that it helped to maintain functional mobility. Student-led one-to-one exercise sessions resulted in significant fitness gains for a group of people with AD, was in-expensive and gave family carers some respite.

- **Relaxation therapy** can take various forms. Progressive muscle relaxation, in those who can learn the technique, can decrease behavioural disturbance and improve memory in people with mild to moderate dementia. Interventions incorporating aspects of touch may also help some people. Hand massage and intermittent gentle touch on the arm and shoulder, accompanied by calm soothing talk, was shown to have a temporary benefit on disturbed behaviour in one study. Rocking chairs can help depression/anxiety, need for analgesic medication and agitation in some patients.

- **Bright light therapy** has been claimed to improve cognition and behaviour in people with AD, though the exposure must be for several hours each day for several weeks and the light must be of high intensity. Low-intensity dawn-dusk simulation, a naturalistic form of light therapy, was ineffective.

- **Snoeozelen therapy** involves multisensory stimulaion using a variety of lights, gently stimulating music, aromas and tactile objects. Regular snoezelen sessions may improve behaviour and mood in people with moderate to severe dementia.

- **Aromatherapy.** Studies have shown reduction in agitation associated with regular application of *Melissa officinalis* (lemon balm) oil applied twice daily to the hands, with lavender oil via an aromatherapy stream and with a course of aromatherapy combined with massage. There were no major adverse effects.

FURTHER READING AND REFERENCES

Arkin SM. Student-led exercise sessions yield significant fitness gains for Alzheimer's patients. Am J Alzheimers Dis Other Demen 2003; 18: 159-70.

Camp CJ, Cohen-Mansfield J, Capezuti E. Use of non-pharmacologic interventions in nursing home residents with dementia. Psychiatr Serv 2002; 53:1397-401.

Chung JC, Lai CK, Chung PM, et al. Snoezelen for dementia. Cochrane Database Syst Rev. 2002;(4):CD003152.

Feil N. Validation : the Feil Method. Cleveland, Ohio, Edward Feil Productions, 1982.

Finnema E, Droes R, Ribbe M, et al. Effects of emotion-oriented approaches in the care of persons suffering dementia: a review of the literature. Int J Geriatr Psychiatry 2000; 15: 141-61.

Gerdner LA. Effects of individualized versus classical relaxation music on the frequency of agitation in elderly persons with Alzheimer's disease and related disorders. Int Psychogeriatr 2000; 12: 49-65.

Grasel E, Wiltfang J, Kornhuber J. Non-drug therapies for dementia: an overview of the current situation with regard to proof of effectiveness. Dement Geriatr Cogn Disord. 2003; 15:115-25.

Montgomery P, Dennis J. Bright light therapy for sleep problems in adults aged 60+. Cochrane Database Syst Rev. 2002;(2): CD003403.

Neal M, Briggs M. Validation therapy for dementia. Cochrane Database Syst Rev. 2003;(3):CD001394.

Powell JA. Communication interventions in dementia. Rev Clin Geront 2000; 10: 161-8.

Spector A, Orrell M, Davies S, et al. Reminiscence therapy for dementia. Cochrane Database Syst Rev. 2000;(4): CD001120.

Spector A, Orrell M, Davies S, et al. Reality orientation for dementia. Cochrane Database Syst Rev. 2000;(4): CD001119

Thorgrimsen L, Spector A, Wiles A, Orrell M. Aromatherapy for dementia. Cochrane Database Syst Rev. 2003;(3):CD003150.

4.9

CREATIVE ACTIVITIES

People with dementia often find themselves gradually excluded from occupational, social and leisure activities or may voluntarily withdraw as their capabilities decrease. This can lead to a loss of control and a perception of helplessness. Creative activities can help to counter this, by providing a purposeful and enjoyable way of passing the time.

Benefits of participating in creative activity

- Encourages normalisation
- Provides stimulation, which may increase motivation to repeat or continue an activity. This can cause a positive change in affect or emotions.
- Enables the individual to recognise an ability to achieve, lessening the feeling of helplessness.
- May help symptomatic control in dementia. Reduction in negative behaviour may become evident as activity becomes more productive, leading to a diversion from self-preoccupation.
- Encourages and stimulates the individual to use memory within an activity. Manifestations of activity (visual, aural, kinaesthetic and proprioceptive) can promote the maintenance of memory, as remembering and attending are closely linked.

General Guidelines

- Try to find something that the individual enjoys. It may mean trying a number of different activities, bearing in mind previous interests and dislikes.

- Don't make the activity too difficult. Failure at the beginning might make subsequent attempts more difficult.

- Be prepared to take part in the activity with the person. The more enthusiastic the helper, the more likely it will be enjoyed by both.

- Encourage choice and don't criticise, even if you feel the person is doing things wrong.

- Find something to praise in whatever has been achieved. Don't try to force someone into taking part.

- Be prepared to devote short spells of time as concentration might waver.

How To Begin

- People with dementia may find that concentrating is more difficult and can require much more effort. To gain any benefit from trying something creative, the individual will need the enthusiasm and support of their family/carers. They must be prepared to set time aside so that the activity can be enjoyed together. Care must be taken to ensure that the activity is of interest to the patient, rather than to the helper.

- Short periods of time allocated to an activity may produce the best results, as interest may quickly wane.

Type Of Activities

Whatever the activity, the emphasis should always be on enjoyment whilst taking part, not on what is finally produced. All efforts can be praised in some way.

- **Collage** Odd scraps of material, paper, magazine pictures, buttons, and any other items that might otherwise be discarded, can be used to form pleasing designs or patterns. Reproducing a picture of a well-know landmark in collage, working from a photograph, is possible provided the picture is kept to a simplified form.

- **Painting** A paintbrush may be difficult to use and implements that are easy to manipulate, such as sponges, rags, an old toothbrush or even fingers, may be better alternatives. Paint can also be blown across paper using a straw. Other things to try might be coloured pencils, pens or charcoal.

- **Papier Mache** Simple items can be made easily from papier mache. Glue is made from flour and water, using a balloon as a mould for a bowl. Each layer of newspaper should be allowed to dry before starting the next. Decoration can be painted or glued onto the finished item.

- **Rubbings** A soft pencil may be used to rub over the surface of interesting textures that may be found on old pieces of wallpaper, coins, wood, book covers and anything with a raised surface. These can then be used in collages.

- **Wax Crayons and Coloured Inks** Fat crayons may be easier to manipulate than conventional pencils. They can be used thickly on card, then the surface washed over with a coloured ink. Once the ink has dried, the wax can be gently scraped away to reveal interesting marks.

- **Mosaics** can be made using various seeds, beans, rice, dried peas and pasta.

- **Flower Arranging and Indoor Gardening**, including planting seeds or bulbs, watering and pricking out seedlings can be enjoyable and stimulate many senses. Herbs and vegetables grown indoors provide variety. Plants chosen should be fairly quick growers. Keeping a 'Garden Diary' can create interest. Pressed flowers can be used to make simple items like bookmarks.

- **Knitting/Weaving** Complicated patterns should be avoided. Simple squares can be sewn together to make a larger item, or knitted garments can be unravelled into balls ready for working. Simple weaving can be achieved on cardboard templates, creating mats or similar items.

- **Pottery** can be a rewarding activity producing a pleasing end product. Self-hardening clay, or clay requiring low temperatures are the most suitable.

- **Carpentry** This is an activity that can be broken down to incorporate a range of skills, from simple sanding and varnishing to assembly of a simple stool or table frame (which can be cut to size beforehand).

- **Games and Puzzles.** Complicated games with lots of rules should be avoided. Jigsaws with large pieces are widely appreciated.

FURTHER READING AND REFERENCES

Knocker S. The Alzheimer's Society Book of Activities. London, Alzheimer's Society 2002.

Kovach CR, Henschel H. Planning activities for patients with dementia. J Gerontol Nursing 1996; 22: 33-8

4.10

DESIGN AND ENVIRONMENTAL ISSUES

The immediate environment of all but the most severely demented patient will usually be the most significant influence on their quality of life. It provides or facilitates both sensory and social stimulation and is therefore a potentially important therapeutic resource. It must be safe, functional, attractive and easy to maintain.

All the characteristics that make a building good to use when mental state is normal become even more important in the presence of dementia. Furthermore, a well designed environment will be appreciated and benefit not only patients, but also their relatives and professional caregivers. The principles are broadly the same in both home and institutional settings.

The home environment

- For patients at home, the surroundings should help to promote functional independence whilst minimising risk. However, the advantages of familiarity may often outweigh the theoretical benefits of rearranging the domestic layout and introducing new features into the environment. A calm and relaxed household routine will reduce distractions and maximise performance of daily living activities.

- Simple interventions are often the most helpful e.g. simple signs and well-defined colour contrasts can be used to help identify objects of importance, for example the toilet door or hot water tap; central heating on a fixed timer setting is preferable to open or gas fires; a gate at the top of stairs and use of night lights will reduce risk of accident if the patient is up during the night.

Creating the right environment in institutional settings

Privacy and maintenance of dignity should be a priority. In residential settings, all patients should have a space they can call their own. There should be a warm, friendly and relaxed atmosphere, aiming to retain the positive attributes of home.

Specific considerations in designing a suitable environment include:

- Single-storey buildings, especially those with a symmetrical, cross-shaped layout, seem to be most effective. Staff can supervise patients more easily and safety is enhanced. Finding one's way around should be straightforward, with clear signposting and good lighting. Partially glazed doors and windows in internal walls will help more natural light to enter rooms and enable staff to monitor patients' safety.

- Use of warm materials, such as wood, is preferable to metal or plastic. Shapes, colours and textures of furnishings should complement each other but vary from one area to another, to help provide cues as to the patients' location. Good natural lighting is preferable to the glare from fluorescent bulbs. Using noise-absorbent materials will help to reduce disturbances from noisy residents.

- Long or narrow corridors should be avoided. A circular arrangement will be good for wanderers, who otherwise can become frustrated by dead ends and locked doors. Ensuring all doors are wide enough for wheelchair access and rooms allow enough space for easy transfer will enhance movement inside the building. There should be adequate provision of hand-rails and other mobility aids. Floors must not be highly polished and patterned and high pile carpets are best avoided. Shallow ramps are preferable to steps when there are changes in floor level.

- Private areas for visitors to meet with residents (and ideally rooms where they can stay overnight) are needed. Comfortable staff rooms to which staff can retreat are essential to reduce burn-out.

- Rooms should not be too large and should be furnished in a domestic style. Choice of colour scheme can be used to influence behaviour. Greens and blues promote relaxation, whereas reds and yellows are more stimulating. Doors can be more easily distinguished if painted in a dark colour in contrast to paler walls.

- Liberal provision of ordinary clocks and calendars and clear signs will help orientation.

- Communal areas should be carefully laid out, with seating in small circular groups rather than straight lines. Conversation and interaction will then be encouraged. Tables and chairs with rounded or curved edges are safer and help to create a more relaxed ambience. A separate television area is desirable, to avoid it becoming the centre of attention. Windows should be low enough to allow a view of the outside from chair or bed.

- Bedrooms should be individualised, ideally using patient's own furniture and belongings. All areas, especially bathroom and toilets, should have appropriate adaptations and aids to ensure dignity is maintained and to facilitate independence. Toilets should be in close proximity and visible from day areas.

- Dining rooms must be large enough to accommodate all residents and some visitors, remembering that extra space is taken up by wheelchairs.

- There should be easy access to a sheltered and secure outside area. Attractive garden areas, with circular paths, places to sit, small fountains, interesting statues and bird tables all help to make the environment less institutional.

FURTHER READING AND REFERENCES

Benjamin L, Spector J. Environments for the dementing. Int J Geriatr Psychiatry 1990; 5: 15-24.

Bennett K. Cutural issues in designing for people with dementia. In Marshall M (ed). State of the Art in Dementia Care. London, centre for Policy on Ageing, 1997.

Brawley EC. Designing for Alzheimer's Disease: strategies for creating better care environments, New York: John Wiley & Sons, 1997.

Calkins MP. Design for dementia planning: environments for the elderly and the confused. Owings Mills, Maryland; National Health Publishing, 1988.

Cohen U, Day K (Eds). Contemporary Environments for People with Dementia. Baltimore: Johns Hopkins Univ Press, 1993.

Day K Carreon D Stump C. The Therapeutic Design for Environments for People With Dementia, Bristol: Policy Press, 2000.

Gitlin L, Liebman J, Winter L. Are environmental interventions effective in the management of Alzheimer's disease and related disorders? A synthesis of the evidence, Alzheimer's Care Quarterly, 2003, 4(2):85-107.

Gresham M. The heart of the home – but how are kitchens used? J Dementia care 1999; 7: 20-23.

Hoskins G, Marshall M. Expect more: making a place for people with dementia. In: Jacoby R, OppenheimerC.(eds). Psychiatry in the Elderly. Oxford, Oxford University Press, 2002.

Judd S, Marshall M, Phippen P. Design for dementia. London; Hawker Publications, 1997.

4.11

SAFETY AND RISK

The concept of people with dementia being "at risk" is well established. It is often given as the justification for management decisions, from the need for regular uninvited home visits, whether by family or professionals, to the need for admission to institutional care. Many caregivers consider minimizing the risk of accident by ensuring a safe environment to be the first priority of care. In general, the emphasis tends to be on total safety and risk prevention, with inevitable erosion of people's personhood and autonomy.

- There is a need to balance the desire to reduce risk as much as possible, against that of encouraging the person's continuing independence and dignity. Everyone, whether or not they have dementia, has a right to reasonable freedom of choice, as long as they do not put others at significant risk. A stimulating environment and positive and interesting activities are incompatible with total safety and some occasional minor accidents are inevitable.

- Good risk-management must include consideration of the whole well-being of the person, not just protection from physical harm. This will involve a carefully considered trade off between efforts to maximize environmental and emotional security and the promotion of individual and community rights.

- There is little evidence that patients are necessarily safer when they are in institutional care than when they stay at home. In general, the more they appear to be at risk where they are, the worse will be their prognosis if they are moved.

Reasons for increased risk of accident in dementia

- Impaired judgement and insight mean that people with dementia may not appreciate dangers and do not react to them appropriately
- Perceptual problems may mean that potential dangers are misinterpreted.
- Deficits of attention and reaction time mean that patients are less alert and slower to respond
- Impaired memory means that patients may not profit from experience and forget agreed safety procedures
- Other physical and sensory deficits are common in old age, increasing the potential for accident. Demented patients will be less aware of these limitations and less able to compensate for them.

Common safety concerns and approaches to prevention
The commonest unsafe behaviours reported by relatives of demented patients living at home are wandering and problems in the kitchen and with driving. The most common accidents are falls, injuries arising from sharp objects and getting lost.

- **General measures** to improve safety include keeping a spare set of keys to all doors, removing unnecessary locks, avoiding clutter, locking up all poisonous materials and installing smoke alarms and fire extinguishers. An alarm system to summon help immediately there is a problem may reassure relatives, though patients may not remember to use it.
- **Personal identification -** It is sensible to provide the patient with some form of discrete identification, such as an identity bracelet with name and contact telephone

number. This can act as a memory aid to the patient, as well as a source of information if someone is "found". Personal information on pieces of paper in pockets can easily get lost and a label sewn into a jacket or coat is preferable.

- **Locks and alarms** may be useful when it is not possible to be constantly supervising the patient, but must not be used to turn the building into a prison. Alarms on front doors should be unobtrusive, but immediately alert carers that a patient is leaving the building. New and unfamiliar locks, or difficult-to-use door handles on exits can act as an effective barrier. They should be designed to enhance the patient's safety, rather than create a sense of confinement. A pressure mat placed next to the bed or in doorways can be used to alert carers when a patient is up and about.

- **Falls** - Check for hazards such as loose carpets, trailing electrical wires, slippery floor surfaces. Install handrails on stairs and in bathrooms and toilets. Ensure good lighting, especially on stairs and in all living areas. Ensure shoes are stable, well fitting and with low heels. Review the need for continued use of sedative and hypotensive drugs.

- **Drugs** - medication may be forgotten or taken inappropriately. Try to make sure patients are always supervised when drugs are taken or use daily or weekly prepacked pill boxes. Ensure unused medication is stored safely out of reach. Simplifying drug regimens will reduce risk of mishap.

- **Kitchen** - supervise patients when preparing food and cooking, especially using sharp or hot objects. Use timers. Store dangerous substances, such as disinfectant, in locked cupboards.

- **Smoking** - supervision may be needed to ensure lighted matches and cigarettes are not dropped. Provide spill-proof ash trays. Discourage smoking in bed.

- **Bathing** - try to discourage bathing when there is no one around to help if needed. Make sure the door can quickly be opened from the outside in case the patient gets into difficulty. Make use of bath seats, non-slip surfaces and grab rails. Ensure no electrical equipment is taken into the bathroom. Make sure hot and cold water taps are easily distinguished, perhaps by painting knobs red and blue. Set thermostat on hot water to maximum of 45 degrees centigrade.

- **Gas and electrical appliances** - make sure gas cookers and fires are not turned on without being lit. Use childproof covers. Consider fitting a gas detector or device to disconnect the supply when carers are not about. Ensure attention is given to turning off appliances when finished with and before going to bed. Avoid saucepans boiling dry - use automatic kettles that switch off once boiled. Make sure hot surfaces (including central heating radiators) are protected. Avoid use of electric underblankets in patients who have urinary incontinence.

- **Adapting to temperature changes** - there may be a need to supervise choice of clothing, especially on cold or wet days. In cold climates, minimise risk of hypothermia by ensuring buildings are well insulated and rooms are well heated. All fires and heaters should have an appropriate guard. Several layers of clothing, including covering for the head, hands and feet are most effective. Ensure smoke detectors are fitted and working.

FURTHER READING AND REFERENCES

Dewing J, Blackburn S. Dementia -Risk Management. Professional Nurse 1999; 14: 803-805.

Counsel and Care. The Right to Take Risks. London, Counsel and Care 1993.

Norman A. Risks. In: Gearing B, Johnson M, Heller T (eds) Mental Health Problems in Old Age. Chichester, John Wiley & Sons 1988; 82-86.

Smith J. Reading around... risk and restraint. Journal of Dementia Care 1994; 2: 18-19.

4.12

ABUSE AND NEGLECT

Abuse or neglect of elderly dependent people by those supposedly caring for them was identified as an issue of social importance in the early 1980s.

- Prevalence is difficult to assess, but a figure of about 4% of those aged over 65 (and a much greater proportion of the demented) is often quoted. The rate may be possibly as high as 30-40% of community-living patients receiving respite care. Passive neglect is reported about twice as often as active abuse.

- The perpetrators of abuse may be family members, friends, neighbours, visitors, professional criminals, or professionals.

- The permanently institutionalised are particularly at risk of abuse from frustrated or ignorant care staff, especially when staffing levels are low.

- In general, the psychopathology of the abuser seems to play a more important role in leading to abuse than the degree of psychological and physical stress experienced by caregivers. Often roles have been reversed and carers are resentful of the need to provide care and of the change in their lifestyle.

- There is often an atmosphere of mutual antagonism between abused and abuser.

Forms of abuse

- **physical** - including violence, and inappropriate restraint.
- **psychological** - most commonly verbal abuse, but also threats of abandoning and isolation.
- **financial** - misuse or withholding of money or other assets.
- **deprivation** - denial or neglect of need for personal care, food, drink, warmth, medical care and socialisation.
- **sexual**
- **pharmacological** - especially misuse of sedative drugs, but also withholding of prescribed medication.
- **forced institutionalisation**, or exclusion from institution.

Identification of abuse
The victims of abuse are often unable or reluctant to report it. They may fear reprisals or feel ashamed and often do not have easy access to an appropriate agency or individual with whom they can confide. Awareness of the possibility of abuse is therefore the most effective approach to identification.

Factors that may alert the clinician include:

- delay in treatment or implausible explanations for injuries.
- patient is withdrawn and appears fearful and reluctant to speak in front of carer.
- multiple and unusual bruising or abrasions, unexplained accidents, burns, fractures.
- apparent misuse of medication, especially of sedative drugs.

- discomfort or bleeding in genital area, or sexually transmitted disease.

- malnutrition, or poor personal hygiene.

The occurrence of abuse is usually best confirmed by discussion with the potential abuser rather than with the abused. Often the diagnosis cannot be substantiated with certainty.

Table *Typical characteristics of the abused, the abusers and the abusive environment*

Characteristics of victims of abuse

- female
- physically as well as mentally frail
- socially isolated and in unsatisfactory housing
- themselves previously an abusing parent, or currently abusing their caregiver.

Characteristics of abusers

- living with the victim and providing care for them.
- age under 50 years.
- male, usually sons or husbands
- history of previous personality disorder or mental illness.
- history of alcohol or substance abuse.
- dependent on victim for financial support or housing.
- poor relationship with patient, with little communication.

Characteristics of institutional environments associated with abuse

- non-specialist.
- fewer residents.
- few trained nurses experienced in care of older people.
- low staff to resident ratio and high staff turnover.

Priorities in management

- the safety of the victim, possibly by removal to another environment.
- active management of physical and psychological injuries.
- help and support to the abuser and consideration of legal intervention.
- action to prevent further abuse in the future.

It has been suggested that screening for abuse should become a routine part of the assessment of carers' needs. There is also a need for the development of national guidelines and local policies to advise management.

FURTHER READING AND REFERENCES

Bennett G, Kingston P. Elder Abuse: Concepts, theories and interventions. London: Chapman and Hall, 1993.

Compijs H, Pot AM, Smit HH, et al. Elder abuse in the community: prevalence and consequences. JAGS 1998; 46: 885-8.

Coyne AC, Reichman WE, Berbig LJ. The relationship between dementia and elder abuse. Am J Psychiatry 1993; 150: 643-6.

Hagen BF, Sayers D. When caring leaves bruises. J Geront Nursing 1995; 21: 7-16.

Homer A, Gilleard C. The abuse of elderly people by their carers. BMJ 1990; 301: 1359-62.

Kleinschmidt KC. Elder abuse: a review. Ann Emerg med 1997; 30: 463-72.

Lachs MS, Pillemer K. Abuse and neglect of elderly persons. NEJM 1995; 332: 437-43.

McCreadie C, Bennett G, Gilthorpe MS, et al. Elder abuse: do general practitioners know or care? J Royal Soc Med 2000; 93: 67-71

Wolf RS. Elder abuse and neglect: an update. Rev Clin Geront 1997; 7: 177-82.

4.13

NEEDS OF CARERS

Most people with dementia live at home with care provided by relatives, neighbours and friends. Just as all patients are individuals, so are carers. Whilst they will share many common problems and concerns, each situation will be unique. Intervention and support must therefore be carefully targeted, recognising those components of a potential care package that will be useful in the particular circumstances.

The majority of care is provided by family members, many of whom are themselves elderly and suffer from higher rates of emotional morbidity than age-matched controls. The hierarchy of responsibility for becoming a carer is spouse, daughter, daughter-in-law, son, other relatives and others. Most caring spouses are wives rather than husbands. Thus most carers are women.

Common Problems

- **Grief and loss**
    - of companionship of a friend and partner
    - (sexual and emotional).
    - of carers personal identity and previous lifestyle
    - of hopes, dreams and plans for the future
    - of income and financial security
    - of social opportunities and outlets
    - of friends

  This grief will not always be expressed 'verbally'. Nor does it go away, even after the patient's death. The carer is actually 'pained' by this grief process and, just as with bereavement, may never fully adjust to the loss.

- **Pain and sadness**. If not expressed and effectively dealt with, then this may be retained internally for many years and may sometimes never be resolved.

- **Emotional difficulties**. There is seldom an easy day when caring for a demented patient and the unpredictability and fear of what may happen next is emotionally draining. Many carers lose the ability to relax and the burden for some can become so great that it precipitates significant clinical depression and anxiety.

- **Anger**. The lack of choice, the loss of control and the day to day indignities associated with the illness can all lead to frustration and anger. If the relationship between carer and patient has not always been good, then the anger can be particularly difficult to manage. There is often anger at being forced into a situation over which one has no control.

- **Feeling trapped**. Many carers feel that their caring role will never come to an end and that they have no control over what is happening. Some avoid thinking of the future as they feel guilt that their only escape from the situation will be the institutionalisation or death of their loved one.

- **Isolation/loneliness** Caring can become very isolating, both physically and emotionally. It is difficult to maintain social contacts and long periods will be spent at home, with little opportunity for conversation or distraction. The sense of being alone, with no one else really understanding the true situation can be intense, a feeling which may too often be justified.

- **Tiredness/weariness**. The burden of full time care ('The 36 hour day') can soon lead to carers becoming worn out. Regular planned respite will help to combat this fatigue and enable caring to continue.

- **Physical illness** Because many carers are themselves elderly, they are likely to have numerous health problems of their own. These may be exacerbated by the physical demands of care. The need for carers to maintain their own good health needs to be acknowledged and appropriate assessment and intervention should be offered.

Determinants Of Burden

- The emotional stress of providing care is in general more burdensome than the physical demands and financial strain. Thus, in a recent survey, 70% of family carers reported that they were stressed, 66% were constantly feeling tired, 40% were depressed and 36% felt lonely.

- Some problems are better tolerated than others. Thus the social restrictions consequent to the dementia and the need to provide practical help with personal care are less problematic than behavioural problems, especially physical and verbal aggression, wandering, sleep disturbance and inappropriate urination and faecal smearing.

Table. *The determinants of burden*

Objective burdens
- patient characteristics
  (physical dependency, behaviour, ability to communicate)
- caregiver characteristics
  (physical strength, competing areas of attention)
- environmental characteristics
  (finances, housing, social network, professional support)

Subjective burdens
- intensity of burdens experienced by caregiver
  (quality of relationship, carer's values and beliefs)

Pathological Caring

Sometimes the caring relationship itself can become dysfunctional, to the detriment of both carer and cared for. Recognition and intervention will help to ensure that the pathological relationship does not sow the seeds of abuse.

Characteristics of pathological caring are:

- a patient who is excessively and unnecessarily dependent

- inability of the carer to set limits when behaviour becomes unreasonable

- inability of the carer to leave the patient, even when adequate alternative care is available.

- difficulties for the carer in becoming involved with outside support agencies, even when help is actively offered

- marked discrepancy between patient's functioning at home and in other settings.

FURTHER READING AND REFERENCES

Connell CM, Janevic MR, Gallant MP. The costs of caring: impact of dementia on family caregivers. J Geriatr Psychiatry Neurol 2001; 179-87.

George LK, Gwyther L. Caregiver well-being: a multidimensional examination of family caregivers of demented adults. Gerontologist 1986; 26: 253-9

Greene JG, Smith R, Gardiner M, et al. Measuring behavioural disturbance of elderly demented patients in the community and its effects on relatives. Age Ageing 1982; 11: 121-6

Morris RG, Morris LW, Britton PG. Factors affecting the emotional well-being of caregivers of dementia sufferers. Br J Psychiatry 1988; 153: 147-156.

Rabins PV, Mace NL, Lucas MJ. The impact of dementia on the family. JAMA 1982; 248: 333-5.

4.14

INDIVIDUAL SUPPORT TO CARERS

Coming to terms with the reality of caring for a close relative or friend with dementia is not easy.

Sometimes termed a 'living bereavement', the process of psychological adjustment to the illness bears close parallels to Kubler-Ross's stages of adjustment to death. Thus carers will often pass through the following stages:

- initial denial and isolation
- anger and resentment
- bargaining and over-compensation
- depression and guilt
- acceptance

It is the responsibility of professionals and services to help carers to accept their situation and ensure as good as possible a quality of life for both carer and cared for.

What Do Carers Want?

Professionals and service providers can help carers by following (or aspiring to) the following:

- complete **information about the illness**, presented in non-technical language. A number of useful books written for lay readers are available

- **recognition** of the carer's contribution and of their own information and support needs as individuals in their own right

- **provision of services** tailored to their individual circumstances, needs and views, through discussions at the time help is being planned

- services which reflect an **awareness of differing cultural and religious backgrounds and values**, equally accessible to all

- **opportunities for a break**, both for short spells and longer periods, to relax and have time for themselves

- **practical help** to lighten the tasks of caring, including domestic help, home adaptations, incontinence services and help with transport

- **someone to talk to** about their own emotional needs, at the outset of caring, while they are caring and when the caring task is over

- **information** about available financial support and practical services, as well as how to cope with the particular problems of the patient

- an **income** which covers the cost of caring and which does not preclude carers taking employment or sharing care with others

- **opportunities to explore alternatives** to family care both for the immediate and long-term future

- **services designed through consultation** with carers, at all levels of policy and planning.

Key Requirements For Services

The ten key requirements for services seeking to develop individualised support for carers have been identified by Levin et al (1989) as:

- **Early identification**. Assessment and diagnosis at a stage when symptoms are still mild enables service involvement to be planned and reduces the burden on carers.

- **Comprehensive medical and social assessments**. This should be multidisciplinary and cover needs of both patient and carer. Interviews should be arranged promptly, professionals should be seen to understand the problems and be willing to listen and a clear plan of action should be agreed and promptly implemented.

- **Timely referrals**. Involvement of other services should be at a stage when intervention can still be beneficial and well before the situation is about to break down.

- **Continuing backup and reviews**. The continuing involvement and knowledgeable professionals is much appreciated.

- **Active medical treatment**. Acute episodes of illness and other remediable conditions should be appropriately treated and the progress of the dementing illness should be regularly monitored.

- **Information, advice, counselling**. Carers want to know about the illness, what help is available and how to obtain it. They also want to be able to express their own feelings.

- **Regular help with household and personal care tasks**. Services which reduce carers' workload are much appreciated.

- **Regular breaks**. Day care, sitting services and short residential stays are regarded as helpful by most carers, freeing them from social restrictions, from giving physical care and supervision and from exposure to difficult behaviours.

- **Regular financial support**. Where available, financial help to offset the extra expenses of caring are practically useful and seen as official recognition of the carer's role.

- **Permanent residential care.** Whilst most carers want to manage the patient at home for as long as possible, placement when needed will relieve the strain on carers and help to ensure a safe environment and availability of practical help.

No one individual or organisation has the ability to meet all carers' needs. The co-ordination of support is therefore critical and may be best delivered by a case-management approach to care. A single professional is then responsible for co-ordinating service delivery so that the various components of an effective care package can each complement rather than duplicate each other. Ideally the case manager will also have direct access to a budget which can be used to purchase suitable services promptly and with a minimum of bureaucracy.

FURTHER READING AND REFERENCES

Brodaty H, Gresham M. Effect of a training programme to reduce stress in carers of patients with dementia. BMJ 1989; 299: 1375-9.

Fortinsky R, Hathaway T. Information and service needs among active and former family caregivers of person's with Alzheimer's disease. Gerontologist 1990; 330: 604-9.

Levin E, Sinclair J, Gorbach P. Families, Services and Confusion in Old Age. Aldershot: Avebury, 1989.

Roberts DJ. Taking Care of Caregivers. Palo Alto, Bull Publishing Company, 1991.

Schulz R, O'Brien AT, Bookwala J, et al. Psychiatric and physical morbidity effects of dementia caregiving: prevalence, correlates and causes. Gerontologist 1995; 35: 771-91.

4.15

CARER SUPPORT GROUPS

Many carers appreciate and benefit from meeting together as a group. Some find information and advice most helpful, whereas others prefer talking about their own experiences and listening to those of others.

Most groups primarily aim to reduce the emotional burden on carers, but they also help to reduce social isolation and can be an effective means of monitoring patient and carer needs. There is some evidence that regular attendance may reduce use of services and delay institutionalisation

Groups may broadly adopt one of three approaches:

- **Educational** : Seminars led by professionals, concerned with providing practical information and advice, so that carers have a better understanding of the disease process, its management and the services available locally.

- **Skills training :** Discussion groups facilitated by professionals, concerned with improving practical caregiving skills. These may include basic nursing skills and reality orientation, reminiscence and validation techniques, as well as relaxation techniques for the carers themselves.

- **Support** : More informal groups, professional or peer-led concerned with providing mutual emotional and social support and adaptation. Sharing common experiences and concerns helps carers to acknowledge their own needs, to get ideas from others on how to cope and to form new friendships.

Practical considerations

- **Who should be invited?** Should the group be open to anyone interested, or should there be some selection process aiming to ensure that those attending have similar social backgrounds and concerns?

- **How many should be invited?** Experience suggests that 8-10 is optimum. More than this means there is less opportunity for each person to contribute and there is a loss of group cohesion.

- **Are patients allowed or encouraged to attend?** If not, some facility for looking after the patient may be needed. One approach is to hold a simultaneous 'patient group', with a programme of interesting activities in an adjacent room. Carers may be keener to attend if they know that the patient is also enjoying some social interaction and stimulation.

- **What professional support is needed?** Will they be able to arrange booking of venues, offers of transport and provide refreshments? Can they organise a programme of guest speakers (e.g. social worker, doctor, psychologist, dietician etc.) Are they available to facilitate the group and skilled at group working? Are other professionals willing to support them?

- **Who will pay for expenses?** If there will be any costs involved (for venue, transport, refreshments), who will pay?

- **What is the best time to meet?** During the daytime may best suit professionals, but will exclude younger carers who are also working. Evening groups are less popular with older people.

- **How long should the meeting last?** One to two hours is usually best. Will the group meet indefinitely (perhaps once a week or monthly), or will it run for a specific number of sessions? 8-10 weeks seems optimal and is not so long that dependency develops.

- **Will the meetings follow a predetermined programme**, perhaps with local speakers each week addressing particular issues? Or will the subject matter of each session be determined at the meeting, according to the needs and concerns of carers on the day? Success often depends on striking the right balance of carer/professional taking time. Carers want new information and exchange of ideas but do not want speakers to dominate.

- **How much time will be spent socialising?** Social outlets will often have been reduced as a result of caring. A successful group will allow adequate time for socialising, perhaps over refreshments after the main session has ended.

- **Who will introduce new members?** Carers are often apprehensive about joining a group. They will be helped by having an individual contact who can accompany and introduce them.

- **Is sufficient support available** to continue running the group indefinitely? Even time-limited groups often wish to carry on meeting together after the initial series of meetings have finished.

- **Is there a mechanism for evaluating the group** and ensuring that it can adapt to suit everybody's needs? Care must be taken to ensure that professionals do not organise groups solely for their own benefit. Successful groups are usually genuinely under the control of the attenders themselves.

Carer support groups will not appeal to everyone. Many people are not interested in hearing and sharing others' troubles when they have enough of their own. Freedom of choice to attend is essential. It should always be remembered that some carers would prefer to have quality free time to themselves rather than attending a group.

FURTHER READING AND REFERENCES

Gwyther L. Caregiver self-help groups: roles for professionals. Generations 1982; 53: 37-8.

Hebert R, Leclerc G, Bravo G, et al. Efficacy of a support group programme for caregivers of demented patients in the community: a randomized controlled trial. Arch Gerontol Geriatr 1994; 18: 1-14.

Kahan J, Kemp B, Staples FR, et al. Decreasing the burden in families caring for a relative with a dementing illness. JAGS 1985; 33: 664-70

Magni E, Zanetti O, Bianchetti A, et al. Evaluation of an Italian educational programme for dementia caregivers: results of a small scale pilot study. Int J Geriatr psychiatry 1995; 10: 569-73.

Mittelman MS, Ferris SH, Shulman E, et al. A family intervention to delay nursing home placement of patients with Alzheimer's disease. JAMA 1996; 276: 1725-81.

Shibal-Champagne S, Lipinska-Stachow DM. Alzheimer's educational/supportive group: considerations for success – awareness of family tasks, preplanning and active professional facilitation. J Gerontol Soc Work 1986; 9: 41-8.

Toseland R, Rossiter C. Group interventions to support family caregivers: a review and analysis. Gerontologist 1989; 29: 438-48.

Wasow M. Support groups for family caregivers of patients with Alzheimer's disease. Social Work 1985: 31; 93-97.

4.16

LEGAL RESPONSIBILITY AND COMPETENCE

The law relating to the elderly demented individual and to those responsible for their care varies widely from country to country. Nevertheless, the principles underlying local laws are broadly similar, even if their interpretation has lead to different conclusions.

Competence

A diagnosis of dementia should not automatically mean that the patient's views are no longer to be considered. However, only competent persons are able to make voluntary and informed choices that are ethically and legally valid.

- Individuals capable of making their own decisions should always be allowed to do so, in keeping with the ethical principles of respect for autonomy and justice. For those not capable of making their own valid choices, the family and professionals' responsibility is one of protection.

- Assessing competence is never easy and patients may be competent to make some decisions and not others. The seriousness of the decision to be made should be taken into consideration. In general, patient's views should be paramount, unless others will be adversely affected or there are concerns about safety (e.g. driving).

- Aspects to be considered when making a decision about competence should include ability to:

    - communicate and maintain a stable choice
    - understand (and remember) relevant information in order to make an informed choice
    - grasp the significance of the situation
    - manipulate information rationally to a logical and consistent conclusion.

- An independent patient's advocate may help decision making. Alternatively reference can be made to a committee set up to consider ethical issues. Neither should merely be used as a way of passing on to others the responsibility for difficult decisions.

- Decision-making ability may change over time, for example as dementia progresses, or delirium resolves. Re-evaluation of capacity may be required at regular intervals, to determine whether competence has been lost, or regained.

Some Guidelines For Management

If the patient is considered incompetent, then someone else must make decisions for them. According to local law, this may automatically be their next of kin, their professional advisers, someone legally appointed by them whilst they were still mentally capable or the courts or the courts' representative.

A number of suggestions can be made to guide decisions:

- the doctor is always ultimately responsible for any medical decision. This should be in the best interests of the patient and accepted by a responsible body of medical opinion as appropriate.

- judging capacity for consent will, at least, be greatly influenced by medical opinion. The doctor involved should gather information from all interested available sources as well as carefully assessing the patient, who should be helped to understand and contribute to the decision making process as much as the degree of impairment may allow.

- close family and friends should be consulted about decisions. They may be able to provide information about what they consider the demented patient would have wanted, had they been able to express an opinion.

- a second opinion is always valuable when there is uncertainty.

A valuable review of legal issues relevant to dementia is available on the Alzheimer Europe website. Individual country reports are available as well as a comparative report.

FURTHER READING AND REFERENCES

Appelbaum PS, Grisso T. Assessing patients' capacities to consent to treatment. NEJM 1988; 319: 1635-8.

Fazel S, Hope T, Jacoby R. Dementia, intelligence and the competence to complete advance directives. Lancet 1999; 354: 48.

Jones RG. Ethical and legal issues in the care of demented people. Rev Clin Geront 1993; 3: 55-68

Marson D, Chatterjee A, Ingram K, et al. Toward a neurological model of competency: cognitive predictors of capacity to consent in Alzheimer's disease using three different legal standards. Neurology 1996; 46: 666-72.

Pesiah C, Brodaty H. Dementia and the will-making process. Med J Aust 1994; 161: 381-4.

Wong J, Clare I, Gunn M, et al. Capacity to make health care decisions: its importance in clinical practice. Psychological Med 1999; 29: 437-46.

4.17

HOME CARE

Most people with dementia continue to live in their own homes for most of the course of their illness. When practical care and supervision becomes necessary, it is usually family members living in the same household who provide help. Particular difficulties inevitably arise when the patient lives alone.

In general, the ability to manage people with dementia at home depends on:

- the level of risk the people close to them (both through family and social ties and environmentally) are prepared to tolerate.
- the degree of control others think it is appropriate to exert
- the price (psychologically, socially and financially) that patients, their family and other informal caregivers are able and prepared to pay
- the local services available to help support patients and their carers at home.

What all patients at home require is regular monitoring and easy access to a crisis intervention service, so that when their condition worsens or a crisis occurs, appropriate services can be quickly mobilised.

By filling a gap, rather than substituting for family care, well organised and flexible community services will help many patients to stay at home for longer.

Involving Community Services

Support services vary from area to area. They may include:

- **formal home care support services**, able to provide domestic and sometimes personal care to patients living alone, or to supplement the 'informal care' of family and neighbours.

- **community nurses**, who may help with personal care, administration of medication, wound dressings and management of incontinence.

- **community psychiatric nurses**, to advise on management of persistent behavioural disturbances

- **home sitting services**, to enable carers to have time to themselves

- **telephone helplines**, to provide emotional support and practical advice as needed

- **respite services**, which temporarily look after the patient away from home, either for a few hours during the day at regular intervals, or for a few days in temporary residential accommodation.

Limits To Home Care

Sometimes domestic breakdown cannot be foreseen, such as the development of acute physical illness of either patient or carer. However, recognising those patients who are most likely to prove particularly difficult to sustain at home for any length of time will help with planning. Predictors of imminent breakdown are those who are doubly incontinent, those who live alone, with gas or fire hazards that cannot be made safe or who persistently wander off and those living with others who become physically aggressive

4.18

DAY CARE

A day care service offers communal care, with paid or voluntary carers present, in a setting outside the user's own home. Patients are brought to use the services, which are available for at least 2 or 3 hours during the day, and return home on the same day.

The provision of day care facilities for demented patients provides both respite and support for carers and opportunity for assessment, therapy, practical care and monitoring of patients.

Objectives Of Care

Different facilities will have different priorities and perspectives on the objectives of day care provision. These include:

- **prevention**, helping people to continue living at home and avoiding the need for residential or hospital care. It is assumed that this will help to improve or maintain the patient's quality of life.

- **social care and stimulation**, relieving isolation or loneliness and providing a place of stability, familiarity and group identity outside the home. It also helps to modify anti-social behaviour and encourages the making and maintenance of social contacts.

- **maintaining physical and mental ability**. Careful observation and monitoring of physical and mental state and appropriate recreational and therapeutic activity helps to promote positive health and well-being. This may include medical intervention and screening, physiotherapy, occupational therapy, speech therapy and monitoring drug effects.

- **relief and support for carers**. Often day care facilities provide the only regular outside support to family and neighbours looking after patients at home. The day unit may also be a focus for other carer support services, such as counselling, education about the illness and support groups.

- **assessment and monitoring**. Particular difficulties can be addressed by a full multidisciplinary assessment and informed observation and monitoring. This can lead to an individualised plan of care that can be easily integrated into the overall management of the patient.

- **providing personal care services**. These may include meals, warmth, safety and security, bathing, toileting, laundry, hairdressing, chiropody, ophthalmic and dental care.

- **resource centre or outreach service**. Day care facilities can provide a focal point for service provision, potentially acting as a 'drop-in centre', a base for meals provision an office-base for community-based professionals and a facility for voluntary and carers organisations.

- **a focus for teaching and training**. The multidisciplinary nature of day care provides an ideal opportunity for integrated training and shared work experience.

Day Centre Or Day Hospital?

- Theoretically, day centres are primarily for social care, whereas day hospitals have a more therapeutic and medical role. In practice the distinction may be blurred. When both are available the more dependent and more cognitively impaired will attend the day hospital, although research has failed to show superiority of one form of day care over another.

- Day hospitals are part of the local health service at least partly staffed by qualified medical, nursing and therapy professionals. Often they are based on a main hospital site and there is thus easy access to specialist investigation and treatment facilities. There is likely to be an organised therapeutic programme, involving occupational therapy, physiotherapy, planned social interaction, psychological therapies and medical management and monitoring of response.

- Day centres are usually paid for by local social services or church or voluntary organisations. They may have no qualified professional staff, but generally a wealth of practical knowledge and experience. The atmosphere is generally more informal and the routine less structured, with often an emphasis on diversionary activities.

Components Of Day Care Services

The key components of day care services that need to be considered are:

Management and Control

- Management committees for individual units.
- Administrative and professional responsibility and accountability.
- Control over transport
- Key workers for individual users.
- Formal communication systems e.g. regular meetings.
- Participation by users and carers in running units.
- Complaints procedures.

Premises

- Location and ownership of premises.
- Purpose-build, adapted or general purpose.
- Exclusive or shared use.

- External access for disabled people : level access, ramps, rails.
- Internal access and circulation space.
- Environment: decor, furnishings, views, garden.
- Main activity, sitting, dining and kitchen areas.
- Treatment and therapy areas
- Facilities for chiropody, hairdressing.
- Toilet and bathing facilities suitable for disabled people.
- Entrance and reception areas
- Staff offices and facilities
- Storage space.

Activities

- Opening hours include early morning/evening/weekend.
- Daily/weekly individualised programme of activities
- Therapeutic activities, e.g. occupation and physiotherapy.
- Medical treatments and procedures.
- Health and personal care services e.g. chiropody, bathing, hairdressing.
- Advice, information and counselling for carers
- Social activities e.g. games, music, discussions, outings.
- Meals. Participation by users in preparation
- Availability of drinks and snacks during the day.

Staffing and training

- Staffing levels adequate to meet objectives
- Availability of professional staff, care staff, organisers and administrative staff, domestic staff, drivers and escorts.
- Visits and meetings for local day unit staff.
- Training, support and supervision for staff.

Costs and funding

- Capital costs: buildings and equipment
- Revenue costs: staffing, rent, heating and lighting, administration, catering, transport.

- Income from charges to users, or official funding
- Fund-raising and donations.

FURTHER READING AND REFERENCES

Alzheimer's Society. Making each day count. A guide to improving day care services for people with dementia. London, Alzheimer's Society 2003.

Alzheimer's Society. Home care services for people with dementia: quality standars. London, Alzheimer's Society 2002.

Askham J, Thompson C. Dementia and Home Care. Mitcham, Age Concern, 1990.

Forster A, Young J, Langhorne P. Medical day Hospital care for the elderly versus alternative forms of care.(CD001730). The Cochrane database of Systematic reviews. Oxford, Update Software Limited, 1999.

Gaugler JE, Jarrott SE, Zarit SH, et al. Adult day service use and reductions in caregiving hours: effects on stress and psychological well-being for dementia caregivers. Int J Geriatr Psychiatry 2003; 18: 55-62

Gilleard CJ, Gilleard E, Whittick JE. Impact of psychogeriatric day hospital care on the patient's family. Br J Psychiatry 1984; 145: 487-492.

Tester C. Caring by day: a study of day care services for older people. London, Centre for Policy on Ageing, 1989.

Zarit SH, Stephens MAP, Townsend A, et al. Stress reduction for family caregivers: effects of adult day care use. J Gerontology 1998; 5: S267-S278.

4.19

INSTITUTIONAL CARE

There is great variation in type and availability of long term care provision for the demented, as well as in demand. Thus institutional care variously takes place in hospital, nursing or residential home settings, provided by statutory, private or charitable (often church-based) organisations. The principles of care are the same regardless of the setting.

- In the past, most institutional care settings were developed with an emphasis on quantity rather than quality. Increasingly the emphasis is shifting to develop smaller individualised units designed to provide greater privacy and to promote maximum independence.

- All should aim to provide a welcoming, familiar environment offering residents choice, freedom and activity, with the support of well trained and motivated staff.

- Good institutional care is designed to provide a positive approach to life, rather than merely a prelude to death.

Entering Institutional Care

Entry to institutional care is inevitably a major life event for both the patient and their family, indicating an end to true independent living. The decision is often painful, especially if the patient does not accept that they are no longer able to cope in the community. Families may also feel guilty at 'failing' to provide adequate care.

Admission to institutional care is most often precipitated by:

- sudden illness or death of the principal caregiver
- development of concomitant physical illness
- development of difficult behavioural problems (aggression, wandering, nocturnal sleep disturbance, inappropriate urination and faecal smearing).

If the move into permanent care is to be successful, there is a need for skilled and sensitive support for all involved. Sometimes a trial period is helpful before definite decisions are made. A review of placement is always desirable a few weeks after admission.

Providing Quality Institutional Care

High quality institutional care is best provided in purpose built, single storey buildings, with adequate open spaces and not more than 30-40 residents of both sexes. It should be sited close to the community it serves.

There is no consensus on the relatives merits of segregation (specialist facilities solely for the demented) versus integration (mixing residents with mental and physical frailty). However, non-segregated forms of provision are probably more successful If confused patients are in the minority.

Key features that will facilitate delivery of high quality care include:

- Provision of **structured activity and therapeutic programmes** for all residents. Care should be organised with the aim of maximising patient potential and encouraging social activities and interaction. Continuing relationships with individuals outside the institution should be actively encouraged.
- **Patient care plans should be individualised** and regularly reviewed. This will be facilitated if a system of primary

nursing is adopted (i.e. care staff working in small teams assigned to particular residents.) This in turn helps to raise staff interest and satisfaction and encourages them to see patients as individuals.

- Particular care must be taken that staff work patterns and behaviour do not have a negative effect by reinforcing patients' dependency and discouraging independence. Investment in ensuring **adequate staff-patient ratios and training** and support to care staff will improve patient behaviour and staff morale.

- There should be **regular visits from specialist medical and paramedical staff** and the institution should form part of the network of local psychogeriatric services. Admission to institutional care does not imply that there is no longer any need for active medical treatment.

- Knowledgeable individuals who are independent of care provision should **regularly review quality of care**. Useful indices of good care include minimal use of physical and pharmacological restraints, encouragement to residents to keep personal possessions. personalised clothing, open visiting, freedom of movement within the building and grounds and in-post training and continuing education for staff.

The UK Alzheimer's Society Person-Centred Care Standards for care homes provides a comprehensive set of standards and key questions to help organisations reflect on their practice.

FURTHER READING AND REFERENCES

Alzheimer's Society. Qulaity dementia care in care homes: person centred standards. London, Alzheimer's Society 2001.

Denham MJ (ed.) Continuing care for older peole. Cheltenham; Stanley Thornes Publishers, 1997

5

SPECIFIC PROBLEMS

5.1

MANAGING CONCURRENT MEDICAL CONDITIONS

Poly-morbidity is characteristic of older people and so most of those with dementia are likely to have pre-existing, concurrent and consequent medical conditions. Their presentation, natural history and management may all be altered in the presence of cognitive impairment. Active identification and effective management of acute and chronic medical illness is especially important in people with dementia because:

- Many medical conditions (e.g. diabetes mellitus, thyroid disease, cardiac dysrhythmias, anaemia, infection) may adversely affect already compromised performance.

- Quality of life may be unnecessarily impaired by an easily treatable condition

- The burden on caregivers is further increased by the presence of physical as well as mental disability.

- Preventive measures or treatment early in the course of an illness is generally much better tolerated and more cost effective than waiting for the condition to become well established.

- Withholding treatment may sometimes be the most appropriate management, but this should always be an active decision made after full consultation with all those involved. It should never occur by default.

General Considerations

- Any acute change in functional ability, continence, cognition or behaviour may indicate new medical illness and justifies appropriate examination and investigations.

- Reporting of symptoms and other aspects of the medical history is likely to be unreliable. Professionals should seek corroborative information from someone who knows the patient well and be alert to the possibility of new medical pathology.

- Presence and severity of pain is particularly difficult to evaluate in people with dementia. Limitation of function, such as mobility, feeding or sleeping, may be a better guide than self-report.

- A practical outcome-orientated approach should determine management. Investigations and treatments that will make a difference to quality rather than merely quantity of life should be the priority.

- Often the development of one new condition may rapidly lead to another and this effect may become cyclical (e.g. chest infection leading to dehydration, leading to delirium, in turn leading to further dehydration, and so on). Such sequences should be anticipated and prevented.

- Medication is the commonest cause of reversible cognitive impairment and risks of drug treatment are greater in those who are already dementing. Both under and over-compliance can be problematic. Drugs should be discontinued if they are not having a clear-cut benefit. Treatment should seldom be more burdensome to patient or carers than the symptom being treated.

- Elective discussion is preferable to emergency decisions. This is especially so when considering interventions in people with severe dementia. There should be agreed guidelines on issues such as antibiotic treatment of pneumonia, artificial feeding, resuscitation in the event of cardiac arrest etc., but decisions should always be individualised. Patients' advance directives should be respected and the views of all family members and involved carers should be sought.

Specific Conditions

- **Cardiac disease**. Atypical presentation is common and electrocardiographic changes may be non-specific in older people. Invasive investigations are rarely indicated. Cardiac failure can develop insidiously and increasing immobility may mean breathlessness is not obvious. Treatment that improves QoL is always appropriate, but secondary preventive measures should be used selectively. The most appropriate firstline anti-anginal treatment is long acting nitrates and/or calcium channel blockers, neither of which are likely to compromise cognition. Active management of symtomatic dysrhythmias, including permanent pacing when indicated, is usually both clinically justified and cost effective, regardless of severity of mental impairment.

- **Hypertension.** The justification for treating hypertension is to reduce risk of long-term cardiovascular and cerebrovascular complications. This may be less relevant in some people with dementia, but all decisions must be individualised. For example, good control of blood pressure in vascular dementia may slow progression. Extensive investigation of the cause of hypertension is inappropriate. Treatment should use once daily preparations with minimal adverse effects in order to maximise compliance. Thiazide diuretics, ACE inhibitors and calcium channel blockers are the drugs of choice. Over-zealous treatment leading to symptomatic hypotension must be avoided.

- **Infection**. Chest and urinary tract infections can develop insidiously. Tachypnoea, incontinence, increased confusion and unsteadiness and falls are common presentations. Aspiration pneumonia may complicate swallowing problems. Collecting sputum or urine for identifying the responsible organism may be impossible and empirical treatment with a broad spectrum antibiotic is often necessary. The possibility of airways obstruction or heart failure complicating pneumonia should not be overlooked.

- **Pressure sores**. Progressive immobility increases the risk of pressure sore formation. This may be reduced by encouraging daytime activity, limiting use of sedative medication, ensuring a good diet, active management of incontinence, careful lifting techniques and use of preventive aids such as fleecy pads and special mattresses.

- **Dehydration**. This can easily develop due to reluctance or lack of motivation to drink, misuse of diuretics, swallowing problems and a defective thirst mechanism. Hypernatraemia may be a useful marker of poor fluid intake. When possible, oral repletion is always preferable to parenteral infusions. However, when needed, a subcutaneous infusion may be safer and better tolerated than intravenous fluids.

- **Diabetes mellitus**. Patients with dementia are likely to be unreliable with respect to dietary intake, amount of daily activity and compliance with hypoglycaemic medication. Treatment should aim at 'moderate' control of blood glucose, as both hypoglycaemia and hyperglycaemia will further adversely affect cognition. When realistic dietary control alone is inadequate, short acting oral agents are best. Insulin treatment requires active involvement of a caregiver, but in some circumstances may improve cognition and general well being.

- **Musculo-skeletal problems**. Discomfort from arthritic joints may significantly compromise mobility and functional activity, without patients actively complaining of pain. Simple analgesics, such as paracetamol, will alleviate most symptoms and use of nonsteroidal anti-inflammatory drugs should be the exception rather than the rule. Intra-articular and soft tissue corticosteroid injections may safely and effectively manage localised conditions. Fractured femur should be treated promptly, nearly always by surgical intervention. Prophylactic treatment of osteoporosis with calcium and vitamin D preparations should be considered.

- **Peptic ulceration and oesophagitis**. These may present atypically with weight loss, anorexia, or non-specific discomfort. Upper gastrointestinal endoscopy is well tolerated by demented patients and is usually the investigation of choice. Eradication therapy for Heliobacter infection may be curative.

FURTHER READING AND REFERENCES

Chandra V, Bharucha NE, Schoenberg BS. Conditions associated with Alzheimer's disease at death: case control study. Neurology 1986; 36: 204-8.

Pathy MSJ (ed). Principles and Practice of Geriatric Medicine (3rd edition) Chichester: J. Wiley, 1998.

Rao R. Chronic pain in dementia: underdetected or undertreated, Brit J General Practice 1996; 46: 554-5.

Sinclair AJ, Woodhouse KW (eds). Acute Medical Illness in Old Age. London: Chapman & Hall, 1995.

Wolf-Klein GP, Silverstone FA, Brod MS, et al. Are Alzheimer patients healthier? JAGS 1988; 36: 219-44

5.2

COMMUNICATION PROBLEMS

Communication is the process through which an idea is passed from one person to another. Ideas originate in the conceptual and imagery systems of the brain and can be communicated non-verbally (for example, with facial expression, body language and touch), or verbally, with words.

In a patient with dementia, the communication process may break down because of difficulty with forming ideas and appreciating the ideas of others. It may also break down because of difficulty finding words to express ideas, or because of difficulty understanding words spoken by others.

General Advice

- Encourage the person to wear glasses (and hearing aid) in all situations in which he would have done so before problems started.
- Don't ask questions while you are running around doing other things and when you have your head turned away.
- Sit or stand close to the person, either in front of them or next to them where you can be seen and heard more clearly.
- Conversations will be much easier if distractions such as the TV or radio are switched off.
- First try to get eye-contact. Calling the person's name and touching their arm can help with this.

Common Complaints

- ***'He says things that are not true'*** Ideas are forming in the mind but the person is having difficulty organising those ideas and making proper sense of them. For example, someone at home may think that they are in someone else's home, that their grandmother is coming to see them, or that they've got to get up for work when in fact they retired 5 years ago.

  Drawing attention to mistakes often causes anxiety, anger or distress and is not particularly helpful. You could sensitively try changing the subject or could say something that incorporates the truth but does not criticize what the person has just said. For example, if the person says he's got to get up for work you could say *'It must be nice being retired. You don't have to get up so early now'*.

  Alternatively, you could try using a 'validation' approach by responding to the emotion which may be behind the words. For example, '*Your job must have been very interesting - I'm sure you must miss it*'.

- '***He tells me the same thing or asks the same question over and over'*** The same idea keeps forming in the mind and the person keeps forgetting that he has already expressed that idea. Telling the person he has just repeated himself is usually not helpful. It may help to answer the question briefly and then try to distract the person from the idea. For example, you could ask them to do a simple task such as sorting out a cutlery drawer or helping to dry the dishes.

- ***'He can't stop talking about the past'*** This usually happens because memories of the past are stronger than memories of the present. Also it makes the person feel safer and more secure to talk about something he remembers well. Whenever possible it is helpful to react positively.

- ***'He starts to say something and then forgets what he was talking about'*** It can help to remind the person of what he has just said. For example, '*You were telling me about...*'.

- ***'He calls things by the wrong name'*** Drawing attention to mistakes is not helpful - if a word is used wrongly, it is usually best to just let it pass.

- ***'He struggles to think of the names of things'*** If you know the word he is struggling to think of, it is usually best to tell him the word - this eases the tension and creates a more relaxed atmosphere.

- ***'He uses lots of wrong words and they are all jumbled up'*** Even if the person is talking what appears to be nonsense, it is important, whenever possible, to take time to listen and show that you are interested. It may help to listen to what you **think** he is saying by using non-verbal clues - listen to the emotional tone of voice and watch body language and facial expressions.

- ***'He has trouble following television programmes'*** For some people the most difficult programmes to follow are those with lots of talking, lots of different characters, and plots that need to be followed carefully. Programmes with few words and no complicated plot may be easiest e.g., sport, wild-life programmes, some comedy programmes or programmes with singing or dancing.

- ***'He has trouble starting up a conversation and keeping a conversation going'*** This happens because ideas are not coming easily to mind. You may find that you have to start up most conversations yourself. The person may be able to talk quite well about 'old times' and you could make use of this. It may be helpful to put together a 'scrap-book' or 'memory album' of clear old photographs of important people and places in the person's life.

- ***'He shouts at me and gets angry with me for no apparent reason'*** Sometimes this happens because the person has misunderstood something you have said or done. Often the reaction passes very quickly and the person himself immediately forgets about it. Such reactions can be very distressing for the carer, but it is important to try not to take it too personally - try to stay calm and let the situation pass.

Making The Message Clearer

When it is very difficult for the person to understand you, changing the environment and the way YOU speak may help.

- Use short, simple sentences. Do not use more words than are needed.
- Speak clearly and give time for each short sentence to get through. Repeat if it seems that the person has not understood.
- Emphasise important words - *'I've made your __favourite__ __cake__'.*
- If possible, point to an object or person you are talking about when you mention them in conversation. For example, show the person the cake.
- Try to avoid questions that need the person to think up possible answers by himself. Also try not to give too many choices in one question - those requiring a simple 'yes' or 'no' answer are often best e.g. *'Would you like __coffee__?'*

FURTHER READING AND REFERENCES

Gravell R. Communication Problems in Elderly People - Practical Approaches to Management. London: Croom Helm, 1988

Killick J, Allan K. Communication and the Care of People with Dementia.

Powell J. Care to Communicate. London: Hawkins Publications, 2002.

5.3

MOOD DISTURBANCE

Symptoms of depression and anxiety are often present in people with dementia, the reported prevalence of major and minor depression being up to 30%. Family members may overestimate the presence of depression, attributing features of the dementia to mood disturbance.

- Depression is understandable in terms of a reaction to the loss of mental abilities and of a familiar way of life and the prospect of growing dependency. Most studies suggest that depression tends to worsen with more cognitive impairment.

- Typical depressive symptoms are more prominent in those with less cognitive impairment, but may occur at any stage in the illness. Atypical presentation becomes more common as dementia becomes more severe, perhaps because of a deteriorating ability to express depressive ideas.

- Patients with AD are more likely than age matched controls to have a past history of depression, suggesting the two conditions may share some common causal factors. A family history of depression is also a risk factor for depression developing after onset of AD. In some patients, the depressive illness appears to be a prodromal syndrome of the dementia. An underlying noradrenergic deficit has been suggested, and subcortical pathological changes are greater in depressed compared to nondepressed AD patients.

- VaD, PD and DLB are particularly associated with depressive symptomatology, but it is less common in PSP and possibly FTD, that are accompanied more often by apathy and emotional blunting.

Diagnosis

- Distinguishing symptoms of depression from those of the associated cognitive impairment of dementia is not always easy. Each pathology impacts on the presentation of the other and communication and memory problems often result in inconsistent and inaccurate reporting.

Table *Symptoms suggestive of depression in people with dementia*

• persistent sadness, loss of interest and pleasure, self-pity, hopelessness, worthlessness, tearfulness
• fatigue and loss of energy
• poor sleep with distress on waking
• social isolation or withdrawal, loss of pleasure in response to social activities
• poor appetite and weight loss (not due to difficulties with food intake)
• psychomotor retardation or agitation
• non-specific behavioural disturbance (aggression, shouting, pacing, over-demanding)
• greater disability in ADL than would be expected from severity of cognitive impairment
• non-specific paranoid symptoms, inappropriate guilt
• recurrent thoughts of death or suicidal ideation

- A National Institute of Mental Health Working Group has recently suggested provisional diagnostic criteria for depression associated with AD.

- Routine use of screening questionnaires, such as the Geriatric Depression, may help to alert clinicians to the possibility of significant mood disturbance. The Cornell Scale for Depression in Dementia allows observers to quantify the outward signs of depression and may be useful with more severe dementia and when people have problems expressing themselves.

Management

Mood disturbance associated with dementia is highly treatable and active antidepressant therapy may improve cognitive ability as well as depression. Successful treatment also reduces carer stress and improves patient and carer well being. Good prognostic indicators are absence of recent major life events, good social network and absence of delusions or agitation.

Spontaneous remission and fluctuation of depression is more common in people with dementia than in non-cognitively impaired elderly people, making it more difficult to judge the impact of treatment.

Antidepressant drugs

- A Cochrane review of use of antidepressants with patients with dementia concluded that there is a paucity of research and currently there is little evidence to support efficacy of antidepressants. Nevertheless, they are widely used and considered to be helpful in alleviating depressive symptoms and improving ADL abilities.

- Choice of antidepressant drug treatment must take into consideration the risk of associated side effects, especially sedation and anticholinergic effects and be tailored for each individual patient.

- The presence of subcortical white matter change or lacunes on neuroimaging is associated with a reduced response to anti-depressants and may increase susceptibility to side effects.

  - Selective serotonin reuptake inhibitors (SSRIs) are the antidepressants of first choice, due to the absence of anticholinergic, cardiovascular and sedative side effects and their once daily dosing. Nausea is less of a problem if the initial dose prescribed is small. Citalopram, paroxetine, fluoxetine and sertraline have all been shown to be helpful and the choice of drug can be based on personal preference.

  - Combined serotonin and noradrenergic reuptake inhibitors (SNRI), such as venlafaxine and nefazodone, may be appropriate when an SSRI has failed, though there is very little published evidence about their use in people with dementia.

  - Trazodone is sedative and is especially valuable in the agitated patient and when sleep disturbance is a major problem. It can be given as a single night-time dose. Excessive sedation, nausea and hypotension may be dose-limiting.

  - Tricyclic antidepressants are best avoided as their anticholinergic effect may exacerbate confusion and they are often poorly tolerated. However, if other treatments have failed (and especially when they have helped the patient in the past) a therapeutic trial may be appropriate.

  - Selegiline (deprenyl) is a monoamine oxidase - B inhibitor and has been reported to have antidepressant benefits in AD and PD. It should not be prescribed together with an SSRI since the combination can produce a serotonergic syndrome.

Electroconvulsive therapy (ECT)

- ECT can be highly effective and should be considered when drug therapy is ineffective or not tolerated and when the patient is actively suicidal, or refusing to eat or drink, or when there are marked delusional symptoms or dysfunctional behaviour, such as screaming. Maintenance therapy after initial resolution of symptoms must always be considered. Post-ECT confusion is probably more problematic in people with pre-existing cognitive impairment, but concerns about ECT permanently impairing memory are unjustified

Psychological treatments

- Cognitive therapy and other psychological therapies are likely to be less effective in the demented depressive than in the non-demented. Nevertheless, more socialisation, validation techniques and supportive counselling can all be helpful, especially in those with milder cognitive impairment, and a generally positive and supportive approach will help to combat expressions of helplessness and negativism.

FURTHER READING AND REFERENCES

Bains J, Birks JS, Dening TR. Antidepressants for treating depression in dementia. Cochrane Library 2003: (2).

Ballard CG, Cassidy G, Bannister C, et al. Prevalence, symptom profile and aetiology of depression in dementia sufferers. J Affective Disord 1996; 19: 1-6.

Olin JT, Schneider LS, Katz IR, et al. Provisional diagnostic criteria for depression of Alzheimer's disease. Am J Geriatric Psychiatry 2002; 10: 129-41.

Rao V, Lyketsos CG. The benefits and risks of ECT for patients with degenerative dementia who also suffer from depression. Int J Geriatr Psychiatry 2000; 15: 729-735.

Zubenko GS, Zubenko WN, McPherson S, et al. A collaborative study of the emergence and clinical features of the major depressive syndrome of Alzheimer's disease. Am J Psychiatry 2003; 160: 857-66.

5.4

SLEEP DISTURBANCE

Many of the disturbances of sleep pattern normally associated with ageing become more marked in the presence of dementia. Thus people with dementia:

- tend to go to bed earlier
- take a longer time to fall asleep
- awaken more frequently during the night
- are ready to get up earlier
- take more naps during the day

Such sleep disturbance is often linked with nocturnal restlessness, wandering and noisiness and poses a considerable management problem to family carers and night staff of hospital wards and nursing homes.

Recognising The Problem

- Particularly in the earlier stages of the illness, symptoms of anxiety and depression may be dominant. There will commonly be associated disruption of sleep, especially delayed onset and early awakening. Treatment should be directed at the psychological disturbance, possibly including use of a sedative antidepressant.

- If the patient is taking donepezil, dosing should be moved to the morning. If sleep is very disturbed, switching to an alternative cholinesterase inhibitor may be appropriate.

- Later in the course of dementia, reversal of day-night rhythm sometimes develops, with drowsiness during the day and wakefulness from evening onwards. This is termed 'sundowning'. Sometimes a late afternoon dose of sedative drug may be helpful.

- Delirium, associated with physical illness or environmental change, may be superimposed on symptoms of dementia. This leads to fluctuating drowsiness, alternating with periods of increased agitation and restlessness. Treatment should then be directed at the underlying cause.

General Management

Non-pharmacological approaches should always be tried before hypnotics are given:

- maintain an appropriate level of physical activity and exposure to daylight during the day and try to avoid periods of boredom (which may result in daytime naps).

- avoid use of stimulants (coffee, tea and 'alerting' psychoactive drugs) after the afternoon. Alcohol abuse will also disturb sleep patterns.

- ensure the patient is not hungry when going to bed and try to avoid a high fluid intake in the evening.

- establish a bedtime routine, perhaps including a warm bath and a warm milky drink before going to bed

- maintain the patient in a quiet warm room and ensure general comfort. If very restless, placing the mattress on the floor is sometimes helpful.

- a background of soft 'white noise' may be reassuring and reduce night-time wandering

- a nightlight may be reassuring and help with orientation

- treat physical causes of insomnia, such as pain, pruritus, dyspnoea, cough, gastro-oespohageal reflux and nocturia.

- consider specific conditions such as sleep apnoea, restless legs syndrome or myoclonic jerks.

Drug Treatment

In some situations, the use of a hypnotic drug becomes necessary. This is most often to reduce disturbance to other people, particularly caregivers who may also be responsible for looking after the patient during the day. The alternative may be institutionalisation. Any sedative drug must always be used cautiously in the smallest effective dose for the shortest possible period of time.

Tolerance to hypnotic effects often develops after a few days of continuous use. Intermittent use, or short courses are therefore to be preferred.

- Zopiclone, is a short-acting, rapid onset, non-benzodiazopine hypnotic that is free of residual hangover. Zolpidem and zaleplon have even shorter half-lives, helping with sleep onset, but they are not as reliable at maintainiong sleep through the night. All have few unwanted effects (though zopiclone may be associated with a metallic taste in up to 50% patients) and they are probably the best and safest hypnotic drugs currently available.

- Trazodone (50-200mg) is an effective sedative antidepressant, with minimal anticholinergic effects. It has been claimed to have specific benefits in the agitated demented patient, as well as in those with depression. Some of the newer antidepressants such as mirtazapine are sleep promoting.

- Benzodiazepines are still widely used, but can lead to dependency and are associated with abuse. Those with medium term effects and therefore little hangover (e.g. temazepam, loprazolam, lormetazepam) are to be preferred. Very short acting (e.g. triazolam) and long acting (e.g. diazepam) agents are best avoided. Paradoxical reactions of excitation, aggression and increased confusion can be a problem and habituation and problems on withdrawal are commonplace..

- There are now no indications for use of older hypnotic drugs such as barbiturates, chloral hydrate and chlormethiazole, all of which have poor therapeutic ratios and high abuse potential. Use of alcohol as a hypnotic is generally inappropriate because of its diuretic action and interference with sleep later in the night.

- Melatonin is much in vogue as a 'natural' treatment for insomnia and agitation, but there is little supportive clinical trial evidence.

- Aromatherapy with lavender oil (or lavender bags or pillows) can improve subjective sleep quality and reduces agitated behaviour in people with dementia.

FURTHER READING AND REFERENCES

Gottileb GL. Sleep disturbances and their management. Special considerations in the elderly. Am J Med 1990; 88 (3A): 29S-33S.

Rebok GW, Rovner BW, Folstein MF. Sleep disturbance and Alzheimer's disease. Aging 1991 3; 3: 193-196.

Roth T, Hajak G, Ustun TB. Consensus for the pharmacological management of insomnia in the new millennium. Int J Clin Pract 2001; 55: 42-52.

Shaw SH, Curson H, Coquelin JP. A double blind comparative study of zolpidem and placebo in the treatment of insomnia in elderly psychiatric in-patients. J Int Med Research 1992; 20: 150-61.

5.5

AGITATION AND AGGRESSION

Agitation is defined in the DSM-IV classification as referring to excessive motor activity associated with a feeling of inner tension. In people with dementia, agitated behaviour may range from irritability and fidgetiness, to active resistance to care, verbal abuse and physical violence. The latter is much feared by caregivers, but fortunately uncommon.

- Agitated behaviour in people with dementia is associated with more advanced age, male gender, later onset of dementia, more severe cognitive impairment, poorer functional (ADL) ability and presence of delusions and diurnal behavioural disturbance.

- Prevalence estimated average about 30%, but range widely, depending on definition and the population studied. Agitation becomes more frequent and more severe with advancing cognitive decline and rates in institutionalised persons may be as high as 50%. Verbal aggression is reported twice as commonly as physical aggression. Aggressive and agitated behaviours tend to be persistent once they have begun.

- The rates of disturbance in AD, VaD and FTD appear to be comparable. It is less commonly reported in people with DLB or PDD. Executive dysfunction is greater in patients with agitation than in those without and neuroimaging has shown an association with frontal lobe dysfunction. Pathological studies have linked aggressive behaviours to more severe serotonin and cholinergic deficits and greater neurofibrillary tangle pathology in the frontal lobes.

- The Cohen-Mansfield Agitation Inventory is the instrument most commonly used to assess agitation and aggression in people with dementia.

Possible explanations for agitated behaviour

Possible explanations for aggression and agitation may include:

- **defensive behaviour** (a reaction to perceived threatening intrusions of personal space)
- **loss of competence**, patients being unable to cope with demands placed on them
- **misunderstanding** or over-reaction to events or situations. An over-stimulating environment may provoke agitation.
- **urecognised pain** or physical distress, patients being unable to convey the experience verbally. A concurrent delirium needs to be considered.
- **fear**, resulting in an act of self-protection

Sometimes the agitation or aggression may be a reaction to carers trying to control other disruptive behaviour, such as wandering or disorientation. Rarely, it may be attention-seeking or manipulative.

Management

Nonpharmacological approaches to management are preferred and should always be tried before resorting to drugs. General rules for effective management are:

- try to identify the cause and treat this. Consider the possibility of underlying physical illness or pain.

- encourage a stress free and unhurried routine for the patient. React to aggressive outbursts calmly, respecting the personal space and aiming to defuse the situation. Provide an explanation of what is planned and what is happening, in a calm and reassuring voice

- avoid confrontation, by distracting attention, suggesting an alternative activity or withdrawing and trying again later

- be encouraging and reassuring, trying to promote independence. Tactfully offer help when needed, but without taking over. Do not laugh at the person's errors and avoid criticism

- do not use punishments or restraints. Patients are unlikely to be able to learn by experience

- consider use of complementary therapies, such as bright light, massage and aromatherapy (with Lavender or Melissa oil)

Psychotropic drugs may be justified in extreme situations but need careful monitoring as they may exacerbate symptoms. Occasional doses as needed (PRN) may be more appropriate than a regular prescription.

- Atypical antipsychotics are preferred over conventional neuroleptics because of their better side effect profile.

- Haloperidol is appropriate if atypical neuroleptics are unavailable.

- Mood-stabilizing drugs (e.g. carbamazepine, sodium valproate) can be considered as an alternative or as co-therapy, when response to neuroleptics is unsatisfactory.

- Trazodone may be useful when agitation occurs at night time, or is associated with depression and anxiety.

FURTHER READING AND REFERENCES

Cohen-Mansfield J, Billig N. Agitated behaviours in the elderly 1. A conceptual review and 2. Preliminary results in the cognitively deteriorated. J Am Geriatr Soc 1986; 34: 711-27.

Eastley R, Wilcock G. Prevalence and correlates of aggressive behaviours occurring in patients with Alzheimer's disease. Int J Geriatr Psychiatry 1997; 12: 484-7.

Eustace A, Kidd N, Greene E, et al. Verbal aggression in Alzheimer's disease: clinical, functional and neuropsychological correlates. Int J Geriatr Psychiatry 2001; 16: 858-61.

Keene J, Hope T, Fairburn CG, et al. Natural history of aggressive behaviour in dementia. Int J Geriatr Psychiatry 1999; 14: 541-8.

Little JT, Satlin A, Sunderland T, et al. Sundown syndrome in severely demented patients with probable Alzheimer's disease. J Geriatr Psychiatry Neurology 1995; 8: 103-6

Stokes G. Aggression. Bicester, Winslow Press, 1987

Tekin S, Mega MS, Masterman DL, et al. Orbitofrontal and anterior cingulated cortex neurofibrillary tangle burden is associated with agitation in Alzheimer's disease. Ann Neurol 2001; 49: 355-61.

Tractenberg RE, Weiner MF, Thal LJ. Estimating the prevalence of agitation of community dwelling persons with Alzheimer's disease. J Neuropsychiatry Clin Neurosci 2002; 14: 11-18.

Tsai SJ, Hwang JP, Yang CH, et al. Physical aggression and associated factors in probable Alzheimer disease. Alzheimer Dis Assoc Disord 1996; 10: 82-5.

5.6

SHOUTING AND SCREAMING

Shouting, screaming or other persistent verbally disruptive or noisy behaviour may occur in up to a third of people with moderate and severe dementia in institutional care. It is especially disruptive as it can disturb so many people. In the community, the prevalence is generally much lower, because it is so poorly tolerated by carers. Indeed, it is the development of accusatory language, verbal abuse and temper outbursts that may often precipitate a referral to specialist services.

Verbally disruptive behaviours may take the form of:

- **Purposeless screaming, swearing or shrieking**, usually associated with severe cognitive and functional impairment
- **Complaining, calling and repeated requests for attention**, arguing and threatening. Such behaviours are associated with less severe dementia and often are related to isolation, fears or loneliness.
- **Perseverative repetition** of a word, phrase or sound (palilalia), muttering or mumbling, which can last for long periods of time and become a major source of irritation to others. This may be associated with executive dysfunction and severe language disturbance.
- **Groaning and moaning**, associated with pain or discomfort not otherwise expressed.

- Calling out because of **fears, delusions, hallucinations or misidentifications**, associated with depression or psychosis

Often such behaviours may be attention seeking and deliberately manipulative. Alternatively, they may provide self-stimulation (such as constant loud singing). All forms can be very wearing on caregivers and others who are nearby and can put the person at risk of retaliation from frustrated carers or other residents. They do not necessarily distress the person calling out.

Problems tend to follow a diurnal pattern, most frequent at night, on waking, or in the evening (perhaps due to insecurity). They may also occur before meals and especially when patients are being helped with personal care activities, such as bathing and toileting.

Management

- A **behavioural approach**, through increased attention, touch and conversation, is likely to be most effective. Ignoring noisy behaviour, or positive reinforcement for quiet time, may sometimes be worth trying. Seclusion generally exacerbates noisy behaviour and is rarely a satisfactory solution.

- **Personalised rather than task-orientated care** facilitates social interaction and stimulation. More time spent on activities, more contact with staff, family and other residents are likely to be helpful. Familiar possessions provide reassurance and a link with the past and may help patients feel more secure.

- **Hearing and eyesight** deficits should be corrected. Patients are then better able to positively interact with their environment and there is less need for them to resort to self-stimulation. Enriching the environment, with use of visual distractions, music and touch will increase sensory stimulation

- Avoid unnecessary and **intrusive background noise** from radios and televisions. Patients may resort to shouting or singing so that they drown out the irritating distraction, substituting sound over which they have more control.

- If noisy behaviour is related to **physical discomfort or pain**, then this needs to be actively addressed. Easily overlooked are unsuspected hip or vertebral fracture, toothache and painful gums, constipation, urinary tract infection and discomfort from pressure areas or skin rashes.

- The possibility of **hunger and thirst** should be addressed, especially in the immobile and those unable to ask for something to eat or drink.

- **Drug treatment** is often ineffective unless high dosages of sedative medication are used. There are anecdotal reports favouring use of trazodone and trypotophan. Antidepressant and antipsychotic drugs may be helpful when depression or psychosis is prominent. A trial of an analgesic may be worthwhile. Night sedatives may be necessary to allow others to sleep undisturbed.

FURTHER READING AND REFERENCES

Burgio LD, Scilley K, Hardin JM, et al. Environmental white noise: an intervention for verbally agitated nursing home residents. J Gerontology 1996; 51B; P354-73.

Burgio LD, Scilley K, Hardin JM, et al. Studying disruptive vocalization and contextual factors in the nursing home using computer-assisted real-time observation. J Gerontology 1994; 49; 230-9.

Stokes G. Screaming and Shouting. Bicester: Winslow Press, 1986.

Werner P, Hay DP, Cohen-Mansfield J. Management of disruptive vocalizations in the nursing home. Nurs Home Med 1995; 3:217-25.

White MK, Kaas MJ, Richie MF. Vocally disruptive behaviours. J Gerontol Nurs 1996; 22: 23.

5.7

WANDERING AND RESTLESSNESS

Wandering or restlessness may occur in up to a third of moderately or severely demented patients. Both are broad descriptive terms suggesting excess motor activity. To observers this usually appears to be non-purposeful and may include pottering around, constantly checking and rechecking, aimlessly walking long distances, or moving around inappropriately at night.

They are especially disruptive symptoms and the demands they place on caregivers and concerns about safety may mean that admission to institutional care becomes necessary.

Possible Causes

There are numerous possible causes for wandering:

- **disorientation** in an unfamiliar environment, such as may occur when respite care is needed, or on admission to hospital.
- **memory loss**, resulting in a failure of patients to recall where they were supposed to be.
- **separation anxiety**, leading to a search for the reassuring presence of a familiar caregiver.
- **searching** for someone or something related to the past, such as a deceased relative or former residence.

- **boredom**, arising from difficulty initiating and sustaining attention on activities of interest.

- **loneliness**, especially if living alone, or institutionalised

- **physical discomfort or pain**, including fairly simple conditions such as hunger or constipation.

- **neuroleptic drugs** (themselves often inappropriately prescribed to try and curb wandering), which may give rise to side effects of involuntary movements or akathisia..

Sometimes, wandering may merely be a continuation of a lifelong habit, a means of using up excess energy, or simply a means of getting attention. Nocturnal wandering most often results from disorientation, with confusion of night and day, or from the person feeling a need to seek information to enable them to feel more secure

Management

Initially it is helpful to review the circumstances and consequences of wandering episodes. This will often suggest possible precipitants and appropriate interventions. A familiar routine will minimise disorientation and anxiety and should be central to any management plan.

Physical and pharmacological restraints are unlikely to be helpful, raise major ethical (and legal) concerns and inevitably damage the patient-caregiver relationship.

Specific interventions to consider are:

- **Personal identification**. It is sensible to provide the patient with some form of discrete identification, such as an identity bracelet with name, address and contact telephone number. This can act as a memory aid to the patient, as well as a source of information if a wanderer is 'found'. Personal information on pieces of paper in pockets can easily get lost and a label sewn into a jacket or coat is preferable.

- **Locks and alarms**. These are useful when it is not possible to be constantly supervising the patient. They must not be used to turn the building into a prison. Alarms on front doors should be unobtrusive, but will immediately alert carers that a patient is leaving the building. Pressure sensors under bedside mats or at exits can also be connected to alarms. New and unfamiliar locks, or difficult-to-use door handles on exits can act as an effective barrier. They should be designed to enhance the patient's safety, rather than create a sense of confinement.

- **Environmental changes.** Use of signs, directional arrows and simple messages may help the patient to locate a specific room. At night, adequate lighting and placing a gate at the top of stairs is helpful. Ensuring an outside garden area is safe and enclosed may enable the patient to wander unsupervised. In institutional settings, circular corridors may minimise problems.

- **Activities**. The provision of appropriate and interesting activities may distract the patient from wandering. They should be encouraged to take part in conversation and to play an active role in the social and recreational life of the household. This should include activity outside the home, including opportunities to go on walks with caregivers.

- **Behaviour modification**. Changing the consequences of wandering may sometimes be effective. Wandering and restless behaviour should not always result in caregivers giving patients more attention and fuss. Rather, more constructive behaviour should be consistently rewarded.

- A **calm and reassuring approach** is likely to be most successful, aiming to distract the patient by diverting their attention to some other activity. When trying to manage a wandering episode, confrontation should always be avoided. Use of reality orientation and validation techniques may be useful. Sometimes collusion, accompanying the patient for somewhile will be the most practical approach.

FURTHER READING AND REFERENCES

Burns A, Jacoby R, Levy R. Psychiatric phenomena in Alzheimer's disease. IV. Disorders of behaviour. Br J Psychiatry 1990; 157: 86-94.

Carlson DL, Fleming KC, Smith GE, et al. Management of dementia-related behavioural disturbances: a non-pharmacological approach. Mayo Clin Proc 1995; 70: 1108-15.

Cohen-Mansfield J, Werner P. The effects of an enhanced environment on nursing home residents who pace. Gerontologist 1998; 38: 199-208.

Eastwood R. Wondering about the wanderers. Lancet 1994; 343: 1237-8.

Hope RA, Fairburn CG. The nature of wandering in dementia. Int J Geriatr Psychiatry 1990; 5: 239-245.

Hussain RA, Brown DC. Use of two-dimensional grid patterns to limit hazardous ambulation in demented patients. J Gerontol 1987; 42: 558-60.

Mayer R, Darby S. Does a mirror deter wandering in demented older people? Int J Geriatr Psychiatry 1991; 6: 607-9.

Stokes G. Wandering. Bicester: Winslow Press, 1986.

5.8

HALLUCINATIONS AND DELUSIONS

Psychotic features of dementia include delusions, misidentifications and hallucinations. They are characteristic of some dementing conditions (e.g. visual hallucinations in DLB) and typically absent in others (e.g. FTD). It has been suggested that they may be particularly associated with disease affecting the temporal lobe and with a neurochemical deficit of acetylcholine.

The sudden development of psychotic symptoms should suggest possible delirium or adverse drug effects. Excess alcohol or withdrawal should also be considered.

Prevalence

Delusions are more often reported than hallucinations, which are more often visual than auditory

- In AD, about a third of patients suffer delusions, typically of theft, infidelity, abandonment or suspicion. They are less commonly associated with VaD, but when present they may cause more distress. More complex delusional beliefs are unusual.
- Misidentifications, such as failing to recognise familiar people (including their own reflection in a mirror) or the belief that someone is living in the patient's own home, are possibly more frequent than true delusions.

- Hallucinations are experienced by up to 20% of patients with AD and may be more frequent in VaD. Visual hallucinations are twice as common as auditory hallucinations. Their content often takes the form of impassive individuals, sometimes familiar and sometimes strangers, children or small animals, such as mice or insects.

- In DLB, visual hallucinations and delusions occur early and may dominate the clinical picture. They may be especially problematic at night.

Aetiology

To experience psychotic symptoms requires some remaining cognitive ability and perhaps consequently they are less often reported in the severely demented. They may sometimes develop very early in the course of the illness, but are more typical in those with moderate dementia.

The presence of delusions or hallucinations is associated with:

- more rapid cognitive decline
- symptoms of aggression
- extrapyramidal signs
- myoclonus
- earlier institutionalisation

Various mechanisms have been postulated to explain the development of psychotic symptoms:

- intercurrent delirium often leads to hallucinations, which are usually visual.

- cortical damage may allow dream activity to intrude into consciousness or remove the normal 'disinhibition' of behaviour.
- the 'pathoplastic effect of personality' may exaggerate mood and personality changes and lead to abnormal

- mental experiences.

- abnormal ideas may arise from the patient's confused attempts to make sense of their situation and environment.

- sensory deprivation might result in hallucinations and misidentifications.

There is no single explanation that will adequately explain the development of delusions or hallucinations in all demented patients.

Management

- Often reassurance and explanation to carers about the nature of psychotic beliefs and their practical management is all that is necessary. A simple change in behaviour (e.g. removal of a mirror, avoiding particular situations or people) may be helpful. Ensuring that sensory impairment is not exacerbating problems is sensible, by ensuring vision and hearing are optimised.

- The continuing indication for any drugs (e.g. anti-Parkinsonian, anticholinergic) which may cause delusions or hallucinations should be reviewed. The possibility of intercurrent infection or other acute illness should be considered.

- Anticholinesterase inhibitors should normally be considered as first line elective therapy in dementia patients with psychotic symptoms. They are useful not only in AD, but also for treating hallucinations in DLB, PDD and probably VaD.

- Neuroleptic drugs may be required when symptoms are severe and urgent treatment is needed, or when acetylcholinesterase inhibitors have been ineffective and symptoms are causing distress. No particular drug seems to be superior to any other, though the atypical neuroleptics may be better tolerated than typical neuroleptics. Small doses should be tried initially and are often adequate to control the problem.

FURTHER READING AND REFERENCES

Ballard C, Oyebode F. Psychotic symptoms in patients with dementia. Int J Geriatr Psychiatry 1995; 10: 743-52.

Ballard C, Coope B, Wilcock G. Psychotic symptoms in dementia and the rate of cognitive decline. JAGS 1997; 45: 1031-2.

Devanand DP, Jacobs DM, Tang MX, et al. The course of psychopathologic features in mild to moderate Alzheimer disease. Arch Gen Psychiatry 1997; 54: 257-63.

Gilley DW, Wilson RS, Beckett LA, et al. Psychotic symptoms and physically aggressive behaviour in Alzheimer's disease. JAGS 1997; 45: 1074-9.

Harvey R. Review: Delusions in Dementia. Age and Ageing 1996: 25: 405-408.

Katona C, Levy R (eds). Delusions and Hallucinations in Old Age. London, Royal College of Psychiatrists, 1992.

Lopez OL, Becker JT, Brenner RP, et al. Alzheimer's disease with delusions and hallucinations: neuropsychological and electroencephalographic correlates. Neurology 1991; 41: 906-12.

Rao V, Lyketsos CG. Delusions in Alzheimer's disease. J Neuropsychiatry Clin Neurosci 1998; 10: 373-82.

Wragg RE, Jeste DV. Overview of depression and psychosis in Alzheimer's disease. Am J Psychiatry 1989; 146: 577-87.

5.9

SEXUAL PROBLEMS

Whilst sexual activity decreases with age, it certainly does not atrophy altogether, and many healthy elderly people who have a partner remain sexually active into advanced old age.

Given the very strong nature of the sexual drive, it is not surprising that when memory of social etiquette, judgement and inhibitions are compromised by the onset of dementia, inappropriate sexual behaviour can so often be a manifestation of the dementing process. It may be a mechanism to boost self-confidence and compensate for loss, or a way of exerting mastery or control over another. Often it seems to be a means of self-stimulation and of gaining physical proximity to another, to reduce loneliness, boredom and anxiety.

Most of the limited research in this area has been carried out on people of heterosexual orientation and it is likely that carers deal with problems of homosexual behaviour with less understanding and tolerance. Most problems with sexual behaviour are found either in men with dementia or male carers of wives with dementia.

Problems involving an established sexual partner

- If a partner with dementia loses interest in sex, the carer may become sexually frustrated and consequently guilty of starting a new relationship if their partner enters institutional care.

- If a partner with dementia becomes sexually insatiable, the carer can become sexually abused and frightened.

- Often the healthy partner may no longer desire their demented spouse because personality has changed and coarsened, personal hygiene and attractiveness has diminished and sexual technique is likely to be diminished. This will lead to conflict between their role as a carer and lover.

- Both partners may be desirous of continuing sexual relations but may be unable to adapt their sexual repertoire to suit limitations imposed by dementia. Problems will inevitably arise when there is no provision for privacy when a healthy partner visits a demented spouse living in institutional care.

Problems involving a new partner

- Two individuals with dementia may sometimes try to start a sexual relationship when in institutional care. This can lead to problems with care staff, because sexual relationships are not encouraged in a continuing care setting, and with children or a surviving spouse.

  The key to resolving the problem is to decide whether the two cognitively impaired individuals are competent to decide for themselves the desirability and suitability of their relationship. This is a difficult area: incompetence in one sphere (e.g. financial matters), need not necessarily imply incompetence in emotional affairs. The aim should be to establish whether the person with dementia is aware of the identity of the other person, is aware that the other person is not their spouse, and is able to state their wishes and thereby avoid sexual exploitation.

Problems independent of a sexual partner

Three types of sexual problem are encountered outside of relationships:

- Inappropriate sexual activity in public (e.g. masturbation or removing clothes in public, sexual advances made towards care staff, fondling or molesting another patient in public)

- Inappropriate sexually-suggestive language

- False sexual allegations, secondary to paranoid delusions, tactile or visual hallucinations, or confusion and misinterpretation of nursing procedures. It should, however, always be borne in mind that the allegations may be true.

Sexual abuse

This can be defined when an individual initiates a sexual relationship with a person with dementia without that person's informed consent. It may occur in association with any of the three previous categories, for example:

- a non-demented husband forces himself upon his demented wife

- two individuals with dementia enter into and continue with a relationship they are not competent to evaluate

- a patient is sexually molested by a formal carer

Sexual abuse may either be missed or be suspected inappropriately if the delusional basis of the demented person's allegations are not recognised. The impact on care and staff morale of such false allegations is obvious. True sexual abuse can result in genital and psychological trauma and, in addition, there are the attendant risks of sexually transmitted diseases.

Management

- **Psychological and counselling based approaches** are often best suited to the problems of a carer who is still caring for his/her dementing spouse at home. If the carer is allowed to express their ambivalent feelings towards the changed spouse in a therapeutic setting this will help to diffuse resentment and guilt and result in the carer being able to go on caring that much longer.

Sometimes problems can be rephrased in such a way that the behaviour becomes less threatening, thus allowing alternative coping strategies to be devised. For example, repeated demands for sexual intercourse can be interpreted as an overriding need for physical closeness and reassurance; if this is the case, then it may be possible to answer these needs by explaining that sexual relations have only recently taken place and other forms of intimacy, such as hugging or holding hands may be successful substitutes.

In contrast, it may be necessary for professionals to support the carer in their initially unspoken wish to distance themselves from their sexually demanding spouse by suggesting that she sleep in a separate bedroom, at least until anti-libidinal drugs have taken effect.

- **Behavioural approaches** are often of most use in institutional settings. Staff education and a consistent approach are most important. Problems of sexual behaviour may be inappropriate in their context and not their content. For example a man with dementia who masturbates in front of other residents may be told that this is not the venue for such activity, and be taken to the privacy of his room where he can continue. Sometimes more pragmatic approaches are successful, such as providing zipless trousers to a man who persistently plays with his penis in public, or separafing a man from a particular female resident who he is constantly trying to fondle. However, whilst a change of environment may resolve the problem, it may merely transfer it to another setting. When the behaviour is to gain attention, then increased contact with family members and care staff is likely to help. Simply providing distraction in the form of socially acceptable alternative activities, such as organised exercise or conversation may be all that is required.

- **Drug therapy** is probably over-used, largely because of the shortage of care staff in institutional settings. The evidence-base is limited and drugs should be considered only when other approaches have been exhausted. Major tranquillisers are often used, though there is no good evidence for their efficacy in this indication and side effects of excessive sedation and Parkinsonism are common.

  There are case reports of successful use of SSRIs and buspirone (probably acting via serotoninergic mechanisms to reduce obsessional behaviour and reduce libido) and cimetidine (through its antiandrogenic effects). Cyproterone acetate (100mg/day) successfully curbs libido in younger sexual deviants and is anecdotally effective in the older patient. Side effects include gynaecomastia and liver dysfunction and it can cause emotional lability and worsen confusion. The anti-androgen medroxyprogesterone acetate (300mg intramuscularly weekly) has been used in the US to curb libido. Weight gain and worsening of diabetes are the usual side effects.

  The use of anti-libidinal drugs is surrounded by numerous ethical considerations, although no more than with the use of any other drug administered to control unwanted behaviour in a person who cannot given consent to treatment. It is considered good practice to decide on the use of anti-libidinal drugs in a particular client in the context of a multidisciplinary team meeting, and to gain the consent for their use from the nearest relative.

FURTHER READING AND REFERENCES

Haddad PM, Benbow SM. Sexual problems associated with dementia. Int J Geriatr Psych 1993; 8: 547-541, 631-637.

Kuhn RD, Greiner D, Arseneau L. Addressing hypersexuality in Alzheimer's disease. J Geront Nursing 1998; 24: 44-50.

Levitsky AM, Owens NJ. Pharmacologic treatment of hypersexuality and paraphilias in nursing home residents. J Am Geriatr Soc 1999; 47: 231-4.

Stewart JT, Shin KJ. Paroxetine treatnment of sexual disinhibition in dementia. Am J Psychiatry 1997; 154: 1474.

5.10

INCONTINENCE

Urinary incontinence is 3-4 times more common in demented than non-demented individuals. The prevalence is especially high in institutions. In people with dementia living at home, the prevalence is about 20% to 30%. There appears to be a higher rate in patients with AD than in VaD. Men are more at risk than women, possibly because of associated prostatic problems.

As well as being associated with major medical morbidity, incontinence significantly increases carers' stress and leads to patients' earlier institutionalisation. The associated financial costs can be considerable.

Aetiology

The frequency and severity of incontinence is positively correlated with:

- severity of dementia
- immobility
- behavioural disturbance
- intercurrent medical illness
- medication, especially sedative drugs, hypnotics and diuretics
- inaccessible or poorly visible toilet facilities

Whilst detrusor hyperactivity (involuntary bladder contractions resulting from loss of the brain's inhibitory influence on the micturition reflex) is the principle cause, other possibilities, such as stress incontinence or outlet obstruction, should not be overlooked.

Assessment

The presence of dementia should not excuse a thorough and methodical assessment. This should involve:

- a detailed history, especially of precipitants of incontinence
- keeping a voiding chart, recording frequency, timing and volume of urine passed and episodes of incontinence
- a targeted physical examination, including rectal and pelvic examination
- assessment of relevant functional ability (mobility, manual dexterity, vision) and access to toilet facilities
- review of medication (drugs predisposing to urinary incontinence include diuretics, SSRIs, anticholinergics, ACE inhibitors and sedatives)
- urinanalysis and culture and tests of renal function
- measurement of residual urinary volume (>100ml may indicate inadequate emptying and overflow incontinence) and, if possible, testing for stress incontinence

Urodynamic testing is often impractical in people with dementia and its routine use has not been conclusively shown to improve clinical outcome. It should be considered when surgery is planned, when diagnosis is unclear and when usual therapies have failed or are contraindicated.

Management
Treatment of specific causes should first be considered e.g. constipation, urinary tract infection, medication, atrophic urethritis, uncontrolled diabetes mellitus, poor mobility etc. There is some evidence that a daily programme of walking

improves daytime continence of demented patients in nursing homes.

Toileting regimens may take the form of:

- behaviour modification, such as operant conditioning, with praise and positive feedback for attempts to toilet or for dry episodes

- scheduled toileting, according to a fixed (usually 2 hourly) or individualised schedule

- prompted voiding, with patients regularly asked if they need toileting and given assistance when it is requested.

Only prompted voiding has been consistently shown to be effective in people with dementia, especially in those less cognitively impaired and more mobile.

Drug treatment

- antimuscarinics appears to be less effective in people with dementia than in cognitively intact patients and adverse effects may be especially problematic. Tolterodine is generally better tolerated than oxybutynin and equally efficacious.

- alpha-adrenergic blockers (e.g. prazosin) may help men with prostatism

- oestrogen creams may be helpful in women with atrophic vaginitis.

- DDAVP (synthetic ADH) can be useful in people with nocturnal frequency or nocturnal polyuria.

Pelvic floor exercises, biofeedback and electrical stimulation are generally impractical or ineffective in the presence of dementia.

Surgical intervention should be considered for treatment of proven outlet obstruction and possibly in carefully selected patients with stress incontinence.

Environmental interventions include:

- enhancing visibility (e.g. painting toilet doors bright colours, signposting, good lighting)
- ensuring easy access to toilets (e.g. no stairs, easily opened doors)
- toileting aids (e.g. grab rails, raised and padded seats, non-slip floors)
- ready availability of mobility aids, commodes and urinals, preferably with non-spill adapters
- clothing adaptations (e.g. longer zips or velcro fasteners, special underwear, elasticated jogging pants)

Incontinence devices

- Absorbent pads and special pants come in various shapes and sizes. They must be put on carefully and be the right size.
- Bed pads and draw sheets are especially useful for nocturnal incontinence, but must not be used as an alternative to changing people who are wet.
- Sheath or condom drainage for men can be useful, but may be pulled off by very confused patients. They must be the right size. A leg drainage bag should be used during the day and a larger bedside bag at night.
- Indwelling urinary catheterisation should only be considered in patients with otherwise untreatable urinary retention, in those with pressure sores that need to be healed, and in a very small number of very handicapped

patients in whom all other approaches have been unsuccessful.

Faecal Incontinence

Faecal incontinence is far less common than urinary incontinence, but is also far less tolerated, especially in the community.

- The commonest cause is faecal impaction, confirmed by rectal examination or occasionally by abdominal X-ray. The bowel should be cleared by daily enemas or exceptionally by manual evacuation and then recurrence avoided by increasing fibre and fluid intake, encouraging mobility and only using a laxative if necessary.

- Neurogenic incontinence may be managed by inducing constipation (using codeine phosphate) and then encouraging regular planned bowel evacuations, by twice weekly suppositories or enemas.

- Pads and pants may provide patients with added security.

FURTHER READING AND REFERENCES

Busby-Whitehead J, Johnson TM. Urinary incontinence. Clinics geriatric Med 1998; 14: 285-96.Ouslander JG, Schnelle JF. Incontinence in the nursing home. Ann Intern Med 1995; 122: 438-49.

O'Donnell BF, Drachman DA, Barnes HJ, et al. Incontinence and troublesome behaviour predict institutionalisation in dementia. J Geriatr psychiatry neurology 1992; 5: 45-52.

Romero Y, Evans JM, Fleming KC, et al. Constipation and faecal incontinence in the elderly population. Mayo Clin Proc 1996; 71: 81-92.

Skelly J, Flint AJ. Urinary continence associated with dementia. JAGS 1995; 43: 286-94.

Stokes G. Incontinence and Inappropriate Urinating. Bicester, Winslow Press, 1987

Tariq SH, Morley JE, Prather CM. Fecal incontinence in the elderly patient. Am J Med. 2003;115:217-27.

5.11

FEEDING AND SWALLOWING

Dietary problems often develop during the course of dementia and undernutrition and weight loss are common, with consequent increased risk of infection, falls, poor wound healing and death. Maintenance of adequate fluid intake can also become problematic, especially in advanced disease or in the presence of intercurrent illness.

Patients with AD are typically thin, with an average annual weight loss of about 5kg. VaD patients generally show less weight loss (and are often obese), but may have especial problems because of motor impairment interfering with the ability to self-feed, chew or swallow. In institutions, up to 50% or more of people with dementia may be malnourished and this tends to be energy malnutrition (low body weight and decreased adipose tissue), rather than the generally more prevalent protein malnutrition.

Undernutrition in people with dementia may relate to:

- impaired cognition, mood or behaviour, leading to difficulty in food preparation and recognising and communicating the need for food
- inappropriate content and consistency of diet
- upper limb dysfunction (motor weakness, involuntary movements, apraxia), interfering with the transfer of food from plate to mouth

- abnormal oral-motor function, particularly absence of teeth and dentures

- abnormal oral, pharyngeal or oesophageal stages of swallowing

- increased physical activity (restlessness, wandering) leading to higher energy expenditure

The nature of dietary problems tends to change as dementia progresses:

- **During the earlier stages of dementia,** the main impact is through the effects of failing memory and judgement. The patient may have difficulties with shopping, storing and cooking food. As memory further deteriorates, meals may be forgotten or eaten twice. Difficulty in recognising and detecting odours may change food preferences, resulting in unusual food choices. A liking for sweet things is common. Appetite regulation may be disturbed and there is a tendency to 'snack', so that the diet becomes unbalanced. Reduced fluid and fibre intake will exacerbate any tendency to constipation.

- **In the middle stages of the illness,** restlessness and agitation may develop and energy requirements will then be greater. Even if appetite also increases, patients rarely consume sufficient calories to meet additional needs and weight loss is inevitable.

  Some patients may start to store food in their mouths ('hamster syndrome'), whilst others do not chew sufficiently before swallowing, with greater risk of choking. Ability to use eating utensils may be lost and there is an increasing need for assistance with feeding.

- **During the final stage of the illness** nutritional problems become more pronounced. Some patients may no longer recognise food and may refuse to eat or even to open their mouth when fed. Others may try to eat anything, including non-food items. Eventually bed-bound, with loss of speech and unable to feed or swallow, patients may require artificial feeding, with all the attendant ethical problems.

Assessment

- Carers' reports of weight loss, ill fitting clothes and repeated chest infections are indicators that there is likely to be a problem with nutrient intake or ability to swallow.

- Larders which are empty (or well stocked by visiting relatives, but little used) are further evidence of poor intake. A reliable dietary history from a knowledgeable carer is invaluable.

- Serial weights (ideally recorded graphically) are often the best practical method of monitoring change.

- Vitamin and mineral deficiencies may lead to characteristic abnormalities of skin, hair, nails, mouth and peripheral nervous system and careful physical examination is useful. Measuring blood levels of nutrients is of limited clinical value.

- Coughing or choking during or after eating or drinking suggests risk of aspiration. Absence of coughing and choking during swallowing means that silent aspiration can easily be overlooked as a possible cause of a pneumonia. Video fluoroscopy may help with diagnosis.

- The presence of dementia does not rule out other pathology and it is essential that the underlying medical cause of any problems is clearly established. Depression and alcohol abuse are both potentially treatable and must always be considered. Oral hygiene and dental care also need to be regularly assessed.

Intervention

The nutritional needs of elderly demented patients vary little from those of younger adults. Ideally, a referral to a dietitian should be made as soon as changes in the patient's diet or nutritional status are observed and alterations to the diet are planned. A speech and language therapist is best qualified to advise on assessment and management of dysphagia.

- **Community services** When nutritional problems first start to become a problem, attendance at luncheon clubs and day centres, provision of a home help to do shopping and prepare meals, or regular delivery of meals on wheels can all be of value.

- **Drugs** blunting appetite or causing nausea (including anticholinesterase drugs) may need review. Review of the timing of medication or taking it with or after food may help. Inappropriate use of sedative drugs may make patients less alert at mealtimes and will depress the protective airways reflex, increasing risk of silent tracheal aspiration. Vitamin supplements may be useful, but appetite stimulant drugs should be avoided.

- **Mealtimes** should be as routine as possible and eating with other people is not always preferable e.g if person is distractible, if person is self conscious or if person interferes with food of others. Also if there are specific swallowing difficulties they can be worsened by distraction (talking, TV, things happening around them). Overemphasising tidy eating habits should be avoided and more time than usual should be allowed.

  Serving one food item at a time, ideally something familiar and well liked may help to minimise confusion. More frequent but smaller meals or provision of regular, nutritious cold snacks may sometimes be a more practical approach than insisting on conventional main meals. Patients with severe dementia may need total feeding assistance which can become a difficult and time consuming task.

- **Food presentation** Cutting food into smaller pieces may be helpful and modifications in flavour and texture of food may make it more appealing to patients with alterations in taste and smell. Use of enteral nutritional supplements may benefit patients who have increased energy requirements or feeding difficulties.

- **Fluid intake** can sometimes become inadequate, especially in the presence of acute intercurrent illness. Maintaining an intravenous infusion in a demented patient is often problematic, whereas subcutaneous fluid infusion is easy, inexpensive, well tolerated and effective.

- **Dysphagia** requires that particular consideration be given to correct posture, appropriate food texture and thickness of fluids. When there is a complete inability to swallow or a very high risk of aspiration with oral feeding, then enteral feeding, using small bore naso-gastric tubes or percutaneous endoscopic gastrostomy, or even parenteral feeding need to be considered. However, long term use of feeding tubes is rarely in the patient's interests.

In the terminal phase of dementia, concerns of comfort must supersede those of maintaining adequate nutrition. Survival is not enhanced by use of artificial feeding.

FURTHER READING AND REFERENCES

Alzheimer's Society. Food for thought project. London, Alzheimer's Society 2000.

Baum BJ. Oral health for the older patient. JAGS 1996; 44: 997-8.

Finucane T, Christmas C, Travis K. Tube-feeding in patients with advanced dementia: a review of the evidence. JAMA 1999; 282: 1365-70.

Franzoni S, Frisoni GR, Boffelli S, et al. Good nutritional oral intake is associated with equal survival in demented and nondemented very olod patients. JAGS 1996; 44: 1366-70.

Guyonnet S, Nourashemi F, Ousset PJ, et al. Alzheimer's disease and nutrition. Revue Neurologique (Paris) 1999; 155: 343-9.

Norberg A, Athlin E. Eating problems in severly demented patients. Nurs Clinics North America 1989; 24: 781-7.

5.12

DRIVING

Driving ability is inevitably compromised as dementia develops and cannot be made safe by modifications to the car, or by limiting journeys to only familiar routes, during daylight or avoiding heavy traffic. Furthermore, poor insight and loss of ability will mean that drivers with dementia are less able to compensate for their limitations when on the road and their mental state may also hamper compliance with family or professional advice to stop driving.

- There is general consensus that people with moderate to severe dementia (CDR stage 2.0 or 3.0) have an unacceptably high risk of accidents and are not safe to drive.

- The relative risk of crashes for drivers with AD of CDR stage 1.0 (mild dementia) is greater than society tolerates for any other group of drivers. Drivers with AD at CDR stage 0.5 (questionable dementia) have an Increased risk of accidents similar to that accepted by society for 16-19 year old drivers and for those drivers intoxicated with alcohol at a blood alcohol concentration <0.08%.

- Each country has its own national regulations regarding the driving licence. Some specifically deny a licence to anyone with a diagnosis of dementia, some require the patient's driving to be formally reassessed at regular intervals, some leave the decision to the professional staff looking after the patient and some place the responsibility on the individual to discontinue driving or inform the relevant authorities if their ability to do so safely is compromised.

When To Stop

- Whether there is any initial period in the course of the illness during which driving is safe is uncertain. Active consideration of safety to continue driving is therefore essential immediately a diagnosis of dementia is suspected and subsequently any decision not to intervene must be kept under regular review.

- Even early in the course of the illness there is evidence that patients are more at risk of road traffic accidents and they may become occasionally or regularly lost. Forgetting where a car is parked is frustrating, but not a safety issue.

- Many people with dementia do not have the insight or initiative to take appropriate action about stopping driving and relatives, friends and professionals must then try to persuade them. Problems can arise if there is disagreement that the patient's driving is 'unsafe enough' to warrant intervention. Whilst many relatives and friends may report deteriorating driving skills, not all are a reliable judge of driving safety.

Factors Influencing Driving Safety

Factors which that may be associated with impaired driving skills and problems with safety in early dementia are:

- loss of cognitive ability, particularly deficits of attention, complex reasoning and visuo-spatial skills. Difficulties in dealing with visual stimuli under conditions of divided attention and of switching of selective attention have been specifically implicated. Mild problems with memory, new learning and language contribute little to driving safety.

- personality changes, lack of insight and impaired judgement

- motor and visual field deficits (in VaD)

- depressant effects of central nervous system drugs

Predicting Driving Ability

Unfortunately psychometric test performance does not always accurately predict actual driving ability on a 'live' test. However, in the absence of specialist driving assessment centres using public road driving, careful assessment of cognitive skills is valuable when combined with other clinical information. Tests should include measures of concentration, attentional shift, visual search and visuospatial skills. There is some evidence that tests of ADL skills may be more predictive of driving ability than brief cognitive tests, such as the MMSE.

After Giving Up

Advice to stop driving must always be followed up. This not only monitors compliance, but provides support to carers who may be seen as responsible for the unwelcome advice. Enforcing decisions by relatives disabling a car (e.g. by removing the rotor arm) or 'losing' the key may sometimes be justified. Removing the vehicle is sensible so that it is not a constant visual reminder of what has been lost.

FURTHER READING AND REFERENCES

Freedman ML and Freedman DL. Should Alzheimer's Disease patients be allowed to drive? A Medical, Legal, and Ethical Dilemma. JAGS 1996; 44: 876-877.

Lundberg C, Johannsson K, Ball K, et al. Dementia and driving: an attempt at consensus. Alz Dis Assoc Disord 1997; 11: 28-37.

O'Neill D. Driving and psychiatric illness in later life. In Jacoby R, Oppenheimer C (eds) Psychiatry in the Elderly. Oxford, Oxford University press, 2002.

Stein AC, Lyons K. Practice Parameter: risk of driving and Alzheimer's disease (an Evidence-based Review): report of the Quality Standards Subcommittee of the American Academy of Neurology. Neurology 2000; 54: 2205-11

Rees J, Bayer A, Phillips G. Assessment and management of the dementing driver. J Mental Health 1995; 4: 165-175.

5.13

YOUNGER PEOPLE WITH DEMENTIA

Younger people with dementia are usually loosely defined as those under the age of 65 years. Most will be in their 50s or 60s. An alternative term is early onset dementia. The old terminology of pre-senile dementia is now considered pejorative.

The prevalence of dementia is about 1 in 10,000 under the age of 45 years, 1 in 2,000 between the ages of 45 and 55 years and then rises to 1 in 500 by the age of 65.

Table. *Characteristics of younger people with dementia that distinguish them from older patients.*

- More likely to have an unusual cause for their dementia
- More often aware that something is wrong and tend to feel more powerless and frustrated
- Often initially misdiagnosed
- Tend to decline at a faster rate than average
- Likely to be physically fit (and so more active)
- More employment and financial responsibilities
- Dependant family members

Such patients do not easily fit into conventional mental health, neurology or old age psychiatry services and present a major management challenge. Key principles in providing effective services for younger people with dementia and their families are accessibility to specialist diagnostic clinics, a multi-disciplinary approach to management, good communications, flexibility to adapt to changing needs and integration of health and social care.

Issues In Diagnosis

Just as in older people, early and informed diagnosis and assessment of dementia in younger people are essential to guide management and to maximise quality of life. Lack of awareness and understanding in primary care and poor inter-agency liaison can too often introduce unnecessary delays in arranging specialist assessment and investigation. Early diagnosis is particularly challenging and symptoms are often wrongly attributed initially to depression, stress or the menopause.

- Potentially treatable conditions (e.g. chronic subdural haematoma, tumours, inflammatory conditions, infection, NPH) are more common, though a reversible cause of dementia is still found in only a small minority.

- Familial forms of dementia generally present before the age of 65, but are still only responsible for a small proportion of cases (probably no more than 10%). Causative mutations are now identified for many (but not all) of these conditions, including some cases of familial AD (APP, presenilin-1 and –2), Huntington's disease (huntingtin gene), some cases of CJD (PrP) and CADASIL (notch 3). Familial dementia is suggested when numerous family members have early onset disease in several generations.

- AD is the most common diagnosis, in about 25-40%. Compared to the majority of older people presenting with AD, there is a relatively rapid deterioration; more marked aphasia, apraxia, agnosia, alexia and agraphia rather than merely prominent memory disturbance; predominant frontal and temporoparietal hypoperfusion on functional neuroimaging; and more tangles and greater loss of large cortical cells on pathological examination and more widespread neurochemical deficits. A large proportion of people with Down's syndrome who live over 40 will develop AD, some 20-30 years earlier than the general population.

- VaD accounts for 15-30% of cases, depending on the background prevalence of vascular disease in middle age in the general population. It includes those with a single hypoxic, ischaemic or haemorrhagic brain lesion, as well as those with repeated vascular damage. It is not inevitably progressive and aggressive management of vascular risk factors is appropriate. In a few cases, there may be a genetic cause for the condition (e.g. CADASIL).

- FTD typically presents in the 50s and 60s and is responsible for about 10-20% of cases of dementia in younger people. Many people are misdiagnosed as AD. Families and community services have great difficulty in coping with the characteristic personality and behavioural changes.

- Alcohol-related dementia tends to present earlier than other dementias (with a peak in the 50-59 year age group) and accounts for 10-20% of early onset cases. These patients tend to spend a longer time in institutional care than those with other forms of dementia, perhaps because of more difficulties with community and family support services, though the condition may become static or even regress if abstinence is attained.

- Other causes of dementia to be considered in younger people include Huntigton's disease, multiple sclerosis, corticobasal degeneration, progressive supranuclear palsy, PD, Prion disease, HIV/AIDs, carbon monoxide poisoning, etc. DLB tends to present after age 65, but may still account for 5-10% of younger onset dementia.

Diagnosis of dementia in a younger person is too often regarded as an end in itself, because the specialist medical services involved in arranging investigations are divorced from those responsible for case management.

Table. *Needs of younger people with dementia and barriers to service delivery*

Needs	Barriers
Early and informed diagnosis and assessment	Delay in identification and diagnosis
Information, advice (financial, employment, genetic) and counselling	Diagnosis as an end in itself, rather than ongoing case management
Regular practical support from specialist services	Lack of awareness and understanding in care services, and poor inter-agency liaison
Flexible and appropriate respite and continuing care	Organisational features acting against best interests of patients and carers

Issues In Management

- Younger people with dementia often fail to fit into any specific category, being too young for routine dementia services, too cognitively disturbed for mental health and neurological services and too physically fit for social care services. Dedicated services to meet the special needs of younger people with dementia are what are needed, but are not widely available. Specific specialist hospital clinics, dedicated specialist nurses and social workers and support groups for patients and families are becoming available in some countries, for example Finland, the Netherlands and the United Kingdom. Internet information and support is also becoming available.

- Younger people with dementia are more likely to have dependent family members and must therefore consider arrangements for their future. Personal relationships come under great strain. Partners may find it difficult to cope with personality change, altered sexual interest, loss of social network, loss of financial security and need to adopt a caring role within the home. Children lose at least one parent and may find it difficult to develop an independent life and feel responsible for looking after both parents (one practically and the other emotionally). Parents of younger people with dementia often find it difficult to accept the diagnosis. Other relatives and friends may become more distant through embarrassment, shock, a feeling of helplessness or ignorance.

- Those in paid employment should consider the best time to give up work. Changing work responsibilities may mean that they can continue for longer. Timely retirement on health grounds should maximise pension and entitlement to benefits. Other activities (supervised, voluntary work) may help to maintain morale and self-confidence.

- Legal and financial matters need to be considered e.g. the appointment of legal agents to act on the person's behalf if necessary in the future (e.g. Enduring Power of Attorney), the management of joint bank accounts, making of wills etc.

- Driving may be an early loss and many younger people with dementia may be unwilling to give up and lose their independence. This needs to be confronted directly, but sensitively.

- Genetic advice and counselling may be appropriate. This may be needed to identify significant risk in subsequent generations, but also often to reassure other family members of no great increased risk.

FURTHER READING AND REFERENCES

Alzheimer's Disease Society. Services for Younger People with Dementia. London: Alzheimer's Disease Society, 1995.

Alzheimer's Disease Society. Younger People with Dementia: a review and strategy. London: Alzheimer's Disease Society, 1996.

Baldwin RC, Murray M. Younger people with dementia. A Multidisciplinary Approach. London, Martin Dunitz 2003

Cox S, Keady J. Younger people with dementia: planning practice and development, London, Jessica Kingsley Publications, 1998.

Health Advisory Service. Heading for better care: commissioning and providing mental health services for people who have acquired brain injury, early onset dementia, or Huntington's disease. London, HMSO, 1997.

Harvey RJ. Young Onset Dementia: Epidemiology, clinical symptoms, family burden, support and outcome. London, NHS Executive, 1998.

Royal College of Psychiatrists. Services for younger people with Alzheimer's disease and other dementias. London, Faculty of Old Age Psychiatry, RCPsychiatry, 2000.

APPENDICES

Appendix I : MINI MENTAL STATUS EXAMINATION

---

1. What day of the week is it? -
2. What is the date today? -
3. What is the month? -
4. What is the season? -
5. What is the year? -

---

6. Where are we now? -
7. What floor are we on? -
8. In which town are we? -
9. In which county/district are we? -
10. In which country are we? -

---

11. Repeat the following words: 'Lemon, Key, Balloon' -
The examiner should pronounce the words at a
12. rate of one per second. -
13. In case of difficulties repeat up to 5 times -

---

14. -

15. Subtract 7 from 100 and make 5 subtractions -
16. -
17. -
18. Each correct subtraction = Tick -

---

19. Can you remember the three words you have just said? -
20. -
21. 'Lemon, Key, Balloon' -

---

22. What is this? (show a pencil) -
23. What is this? (show a watch) -

24. Repeat the following 'No ifs, ands or buts' -

Follow a three-stage command:
25. 'Take this piece of paper, -
26. fold it in half, -
27. and put it on the floor'. -

(Maximum 3 points)

---

28. Read and obey what is written on this piece of paper

('Close your eyes') -

---

29. Write a sentence of your choice on this piece of paper -

---

30. Copy this drawing on a piece of paper -

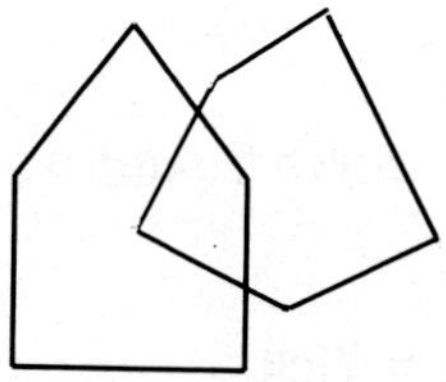

TOTAL [|]

Reference : Folstein MF, Folstein SE, McHugh PR. Minimental State. A practical method for grading the cognitive state of patients for clinician. J Psychiat Res. 1975; 12: 189-98.

Appendix II : HACHINSKI ISCHAEMIC SCORE

Abrupt onset	2
Stepwise deterioration	1
Fluctuating course	2
Nocturnal confusion	1
Relative preservation of personality	1
Depression	1
Somatic complaints	1
Emotional incontinence	1
History of hypertension	1
History of strokes	2
Evidence of associated atherosclerosis	1
Focal neurological symptoms	2
Focal neurological signs	2

TOTAL ☐☐

Score: 0-4 Alzheimer's disease;
5,6 Mixed Alzheimer's/vascular disease;
7+ Multi infarct dementia.

Reference: Hachinski VC, et al. Cerebral blood flow in dementia. Arch Neurol 1975; 32: 632-7

Appendix III : GERIATRIC DEPRESSION SCALE (GDS-15)

1. Are you basically satisfied with your life? Yes/**NO**
2. Have you dropped many of your activities and interests? **YES**/No
3. Do you feel that your life is empty? **YES**/No
4. Do you often get bored? **YES**/No
5. Are you in good spirits most of the time? yes/**NO**
6. Are you afraid that something bad is going to happen to you? **YES**/No
7. Do you feel happy most of the time? yes/**NO**
8. Do you often feel helpless? **YES**/No
9. Do you prefer to stay at home, rather than going out and doing new things? **YES**/No
10. Do you feel you have problems with memory more than most? **YES**/No

11. Do you think it is wonderful to be alive now? yes/**NO**

12. Do you feel pretty worthless the way you are now? **YES**/No

13. Do you feel full of energy? yes/**NO**

14. Do you feel that your situation is hopeless? **YES**/No

15. Do you think that most people are better off then you are? **YES**/No

TOTAL (of answers in capitals) ☐

Score: >/=5 suggests possible depression

Reference: Sheik J, Yesavage JA, Geriatric Depression Scale : recent evidence and development of a shorter version. In : Brink TL (ed) Clinical Gerontology : a guide to assessment and intervention. New York, Haworth Press, 1986.

Appendix IV : DSM-IV DIAGNOSTIC CRITERIA FOR DEMENTIA

A. The development of multiple cognitive deficits manifested by:

1) memory impairment (inability to learn new information and to recall previously learned information) AND

2) at least one of the following cognitive disturbances:
   a) aphasia (language disturbance)
   b) apraxia (inability to carry out motor activities despite intact motor function)
   c) agnosia (failure to recognise or identify objects despite intact sensory function)
   d) disturbance in executive functioning (i.e. planning, organising sequencing, abstracting)

B. The course is characterised by gradual onset and continuing cognitive decline

C. The cognitive deficits cause significant impairment in social or occupational functioning and represent a significant decline from a previous level of functioning.

E. The deficits do not occur exclusively during the course of Delirium

F. Not better accounted for by another Axis I disorder (e.g. Major Depressive Disorders, Schizophrenia).

Reference: American Psychiatric Association. Diagnostic & Statistical Mannual of Mental Disorders. Fourth Edition (DSM-IV). Washington DC 1994.

Appendix V : NINCDS-ADRDA CRITERIA FOR PROBABLE ALZHEIMER'S DISEASE

1. Criteria for diagnosis include:

(a) dementia established by clinical examination and documented by the Mini-Mental Test, Blessed Dementia Scale or some similar examination and confirmed by neuropsychological tests.

(b) deficits in two or more areas of cognition

(c) progressive worsening of memory and other cognitive functions

(d) no disturbance of consciousness

(e) onset between ages 40 & 90, most often after 65

(f) absence of systemic disorders or other brain diseases that could account for the progressive deficits in memory and cognition

2. The diagnosis is supported by:

(a) progressive deterioration of specific cognitive functions such as language (aphasia), motor skills (apraxia), and perception (agnosia).

(b) impaired activities of daily living and altered patterns of behaviour

(c) family history of similar disorders, particularly if confirmed neuropathologically

(d) laboratory results of normal lumbar puncture as evaluated by standard techniques, normal pattern or non-specific changes in EEG, such as increased slow-wave activity and evidence of cerebral atrophy on CT with progression documented by serial observation.

3. Other clinical features consistent with the diagnosis, after exclusion of causes of dementia other than Alzheimer's disease include:

(a) plateaus in the course of illness progression

(b) associated symptoms of depression, insomnia, incontinence, delusions, illusions, hallucinations, catastrophic verbal, emotional or physical outbursts, sexual disorders, and weight loss

(c) other neurological abnormalities in some patients, especially with more advanced disease and inclusion motor signs such as increased muscle tone, myoclonus, or gait disorder

(d) seizures in advanced disease

(e) CT normal for age

Reference: McKhann G, et al. Clinial diagnosis of Alzheimer disease: Report of the NINCDS-ADRDA Work Group under the auspices of Department of Health & Human Services Task Force on Alzheimer's Disease. Neurology 1984 : 34; 939-944.

Appendix VI : CONSENSUS CRITERIA FOR CLINICAL DIAGNOSIS OF DEMENTIA WITH LEWY BODIES

1. The central feature is progressive cognitive decline amounting to **dementia**; prominent or persistent memory deficit may not occur in early stages; deficits on tests of attention, fronto-cortical skills and visuospatial ability may be especially prominent

2. Two of the following core features are required for a probable, and one for a possible diagnosis of DLB:

   - **Fluctuating cognition** with pronounced variation in attention and alertness

   - **Recurrent visual hallucinations** that arc typically well formed and detailed

   - Spontaneous motor features of **Parkinsonism**

3. Features supportive of the diagnosis are:

   - Repeated falls
   - Syncope or transient loss of consciousness
   - Neuroleptic hypersensitivity
   - Systematized delusions
   - Non-visual hallucinations
   - Depression *
   - REM Sleep Behaviour Disorder *

4. DLB is less likely in the presence of:

- Stroke disease, revealed by focal neurological signs or brain imaging
- Evidence of any other physical or brain illness that may account for the clinical picture

* *added as possible additional supportive features at Second International Meeting (McKeith et al.Neurology 1999;53:902-5)*

Reference: McKeith IG, Galasko D, Kosaka K, et al. Consensus Guidelines for the clinical and pathological diagnosis of dementia with Lewy bodies (DLB): report of the consortium on DLB international workshop. Neurology 1996; 47: 1113-24.

Appendix VII : LUND/ MANCHESTER CRITERIA FOR FRONTO-TEMPORAL DEMENTIA

Core diagnostic features include:

Behavioral disorder

- Insidious onset and slow progression
- Early loss of personal awareness
- Early loss of social awareness
- Early signs of disinhibition
- Mental rigidity and inflexibility
- Hyperorality
- Stereotyped and perseverative behavior
- Utilization behavior
- Distractability, impulsivity, and impersistence
- Early loss of insight

Affective symptoms

- Depression, anxiety, excessive sentimentality, suicidal ideation, delusion
- Hypochondriasis, bizarre somatic preoccupation
- Emotional unconcern
- Amimia (aspontaneity)

Speech disorder

- Progressive reduction of speech
- Stereotypy of speech
- Echolalia and perseveration
- Late mutism

Spatial orientation and praxis preserved

Physical signs

- Early primitive reflexes
- Early incontinence
- Late akinesia, rigidity, tremor
- Low and labile blood pressure

Investigations

- Electroencephalogram: normal
- Brain imaging: frontal or anterior temporal changes or both
- Neuropsychology: fail frontal lobe tests

Supportive diagnostic features include:

- Onset before age 65
- Positive family history of similar disorder in first degree relative
- Motor neuron disease

Reference Adapted from Brun A, Englund L, Gustafson L, et al Consensus statement: clinical and neuropathological criteria for frontotemporal dementia. J Neurol Neurosurg Psychiatry 1994; 57: 416

Appendix VIII : NINDS-AIREN CRITERIA FOR CLINICAL DIAGNOSIS OF PROBABLE VASCULAR DEMENTIA

I. The criteria for the clinical diagnosis of probable vascular dementia include all of the following:

(1) ***Dementia*** defined by cognitive decline from a previously higher level of functioning and manifested by impairment of memory and of two or more cognitive domains (orientation, attention, language, visuospatial functions, executive functions, motor control, and praxis), preferably established by clinical examination and documented by neuropsychological testing.

Deficits should be severe enough to interfere with activities of daily living not due to physical effects of stroke alone.

Exclusion criteria: cases with disturbance of consciousness, delirium, psychosis, severe aphasia, or major sensorimotor impairment precluding neuropsychological testing.

Also excluded are systemic disorders or other brain diseases (such as Alzheimer's Disease) that in and of themselves could account for deficits in memory and cognition

(2) ***Cerebrovascular disease***, defined by the presence of focal signs on neurologic examination, such as hemiparesis, lower facial weakness, Babinski sign,

sensory deficit, hemianopia, and dysarthria consistent with stroke (with or without history of stroke) and

Evidence of relevant cerebrovascular disease by brain imaging (CT or MRI) including multiple large-vessel infarcts or a single strategically placed infarct (angular gyrus, thalamus, basal forebrain, or posterior cerebral artery or anterior cerebral artery territories), as well as multiple basal ganglia and white matter lacunes or extensive periventricular white matter lesions, or combination thereof.

(3) A relationship between the above two disorders, manifested or inferred by the presence of one or more of the following

(a)onset of dementia within 3 months following a recognised stroke:

(b) abrupt deterioration in cognitive functions; or fluctuating, stepwise progression of cognitive deficits.

II. Clinical features consistent with the diagnosis of probable vascular dementia include the following:

(a) Early presence of a gait disturbance (small-step gait or marche a petits pas, or magnetic, apraxic-ataxic or parkinsonian gait);

(b) history of unsteadiness and frequent, unprovoked falls;

(c) early urinary frequency, urgency, and other urinary symptoms not explained by urologic disease;

(d) pseudobulbar palsy;

(e) personality and mood changes, abulia, depression, emotional incontinence, or other subcortical deficits including psychomotor retardation and abnormal executive function.

III. Features that make the diagnosis of vascular dementia uncertain or unlikely include

(a) early onset of memory deficit and progressive worsening of memory and other cognitive functions such as language (transcortical sensory aphasia), motor skills (apraxia), and perception (agnosia), in the absence of corresponding focal lesions on brain imaging;

(b) absence of focal neurologic signs, other than cognitive disturbance;

(c) absence of cerebrovascular lesions on brain CT or MRI.

Reference: Roman GC, et al. Vascular dementia: Diagnostic criteria for research studies. Neurology 1993 43; 250-260.

Appendix IX : CLINICAL GUIDELINES

A range of authoritative guidelines on assessment, diagnosis and management of dementia and related issues have been published by governmental, professional and patient organisations in North America and Europe. They can become outdated very rapidly, but serve as a basis for good practice.

A comprehensive review of guidelines is available in : Burns A, Denning T, Lawlor B. 'Clinical Guidelines in Old Age Psychiatry'. London: Martin Dunitz, 2001.

Useful websites are:

- National Electronic Library for Health Guidelines Finder (www.nelh.nhs.uk/guidelinesfinder)
- National Guideline Clearing House (www.guideline.gov)

Among the most authoritative guidelines are:

Early Detection Of Dementia And Mild Cognitive Impairment : Peterson RC, Stevens JC, Ganguli M, et al. Practice Parameter: Early detection of Dementia: mild cognitive impairment (an Evidence-based Review): report of the Quality Standards Subcommittee of the American Academy of Neurology. Neurology 2001; 56: 1133-42

Screening For Dementia : U.S. Preventive Services Task Force. Screening for dementia: recommendation and rationale. Ann Intern Med 2003 ;138:925-6

Predictive Testing For Alzheimer's Disease : Consensus statement on predictive testing for Alzheimer's disease. Alz Dis Assoc Disord 1995; 94: 182-7

Molecular And Biochemical Markers Of Alzheimer's Disease : Consensus Report of the Working Group on: 'Molecular and Biochemical Markers of Alzheimer's Disease'. Neurobiol Aging 1998; 19: 109-16.

Genetic Testing For Alzheimer's Disease : Post SG, Whitehouse P, Binstock RH, et al. Consensus statement. The clinical introduction of genetic testing for Alzheimer's disease: an ethical perspective. JAMA 1997; 277: 832-6.

Diagnosis Of Alzheimer's Disease : McKhann G, Drachman D, Folstein M, Katzman R, Price D, Stadlan EM. Clinical diagnosis of Alzheimer's disease: report of the NINCDS-ADRDA Work Group under the auspices of Department of Health and Human Services Task Force on Alzheimer's Disease. Neurology. 1984;34:939-44.

Clinical And Neuropsychological Assessment Of Alzheimer's Disease : Morris JC, Heyman A, Mohs RC, et al. Consortium to Establish a Registry for Alzheimer's Disease (CERAD) Part I: Clinical and neuropsychological assessment of Alzheimer's disease. Neurology 1989; 39: 1159-65

Diagnosis And Management Of Alzheimer's Disease And Other Dementia : Waldemar G, Dubois B, Emre M, et al. Diagnosis and management of Alzheimer's disease and other disorders associated with dementia. The role of neurologists in Europe. European federation of Neurological Societies. Eur J Neurology 20000; 7: 133-44.

Cholinesterase Inhibitor Drugs For Alzheimer's Disease : National Institute for Clinical Excellence (NICE). Guidance on the use of donepezil, rivastigmine and galantamine for the treatment of Alzheimer's disease. Technology Appraisal Guidance No. 19. (www.nice.org.uk)

Diagnosis Of Frontotemporal Dementia : Neary D, Snowden JS, Gustafson L, Passant U, Stuss D, Black S, Freedman M, Kertesz A, Robert PH, Albert M, Boone K, Miller BL, Cummings J, Benson DF. Frontotemporal lobar degeneration:

a consensus on clinical diagnostic criteria. Neurology. 1998;5:1546-54.

Diagnosis Of Frontotemporal Dementia : McKhann GM, Albert MS, Grossman M, Miller B, Dickson D, Trojanowski JQ; Work Group on Frontotemporal Dementia and Pick's Disease. Clinical and pathological diagnosis of frontotemporal dementia: report of the Work Group on Frontotemporal Dementia and Pick's Disease. Arch Neurol. 2001;58:1803-9.

Diagnosis Of Vascular Dementia : Chui HC, Victoroff JI, Margolin D, Jagust W, Shankle R, Katzman R. Criteria for the diagnosis of ischemic vascular dementia proposed by the State of California Alzheimer's Disease Diagnostic and Treatment Centers. Neurology. 1992 ;42:473-80.

Diagnosis Of Vascular Dementia : Roman GC, Tatemichi TK, Erkinjuntti T, Cummings JL, Masdeu JC, Garcia JH, Amaducci L, Orgogozo JM, Brun A, Hofman A, et al. Vascular dementia: diagnostic criteria for research studies. Report of the NINDS-AIREN International Workshop. Neurology. 1993;43:250-60.

Diagnosis Of Dementia With Lewy Bodies : McKeith IG, Galasko D, Kosaka K, et al. Consensus guidelines for the clinical and pathologic diagnosis of dementia with Lewy bodies (DLB): report of the consortium on DLB international workshop. Neurology. 1996 ;47:1113-24.

Dementia Diagnosis And Assessment : Knopman DS, DeKosky ST, Cummings JL, et al. Practice Parameter: Diagnosis of Dementia (an Evidence-based Review): report of the Quality Standards Subcommittee of the American Academy of Neurology. Neurology 2001; 56: 1143-53

Primary Care Management Of Dementia : Eccles M, Clarke J, Livingstone M, et al. North of England evidence-based guidelines development project: guideline for the primary care management of dementia. BMJ 1998; 317: 802-8.

Management Of Behavioural And Psychological Aspects Of Dementia : Scottish Inter-Collegiate Guidelines Network (SIGN). Royal College of Physicians, Edinburgh 1998. (www.show.scot.nhs.uk/sign/pdf/sign22.pdf)

Management Of Agitation : Howard R, Ballard C, O'Brien J, et al. Guidelines for the management of agitation in dementia. Int J Geriatr Psychiatry. 2001;16:714-7.

Management Of Dementia : Doody RS, Steven JC, Beck C, et al. Practice Parameter: Management of Dementia (an Evidence-based Review): report of the Quality Standards Subcommittee of the American Academy of Neurology. Neurology 2001; 56: 1154-66

Risk Of Driving And Alzheimer's Disease : Dubinsky RM, Stein AC, Lyons K.. Practice Parameter: risk of driving and Alzheimer's disease (an Evidence-based Review): report of the Quality Standards Subcommittee of the American Academy of Neurology. Neurology 2000; 54: 2205-11

Neuropathological Assessment Of Alzheimer's Disease : Mirra SS, Heyman A, McKeel DW, et al. Consortium to Establish a Registry for Alzheimer's Disease (CERAD) PartII: Standardization of the neuropathological assessment of Alzheimer's disease. Neurology 1991; 41: 479-86.

Dementia Among Adults With Intellectual Disorders: Janicki MP, Heller T, Seltzer GB, Et Al. Practice Guidelines For The Clinical Assessment And Care Management Of Alzheimer's Disease And Other Dementias Among Adults With Intellectual Disability. J Intellectual Dis Research 1996; 40: 374-82.

Dementia Among Adults With Intellectual Disorders: Wilkinson H, Janicki MP; Edinburgh Working Group On Dementia Care Practices (EWGDCP). The Edinburgh Principles With Accompanying Guidelines And Recommendations. J Intellect Disabil Res. 2002;46:279-84

Appendix X : WEBSITES

Most national Alzheimer organisations have their own websites with relevant locally orientated materials and links.

A selection of website resources and useful links is listed below.

A list of websites containing information on various aspects of dementia in languages other than English (from Arabic to Welsh) is available on the Alzheimer Disease International website **(http://www.alz.co.uk)**

UK Alzheimer Society
http://www.alzheimers.org.uk

UK-based dementia research centre
http://www.kingshill-research.org

US-based site with comprehensive carer information
http://www.agenet.com/alzheimer_links.html

Dementia Advice and Support Learning Network
http://www.mhilli.org/network/network.htm

Lewy-Net – information on dementia with Lewy bodies
http://www.nottingham.ac.uk/pathology/lewy/lewyhome.html

Alzheimer's Association, Australia site
http://www.alzheimers.org.au

Alzheimer Society of Canada (in English and French)
http://www.alzheimer.ca

Alzheimer's Disease Review
http://www.coa.uky.edu/ADReview/

Centre for Social Research in Dementia
http://www.stir.ac.uk/appsocsci/CSRD/research

Cochrane Library
http://www.cochranelibrary.com/cochrane

Dementia Advocacy and Support
http:www.dasninternational.org

Dementia Services Development Centre, Bristol
http://www.dementia-voice.org.uk

Dementia web
http://dementia.ion.ucl.ac.uk/dementia

National Electronic Library for Health
http://www.nelh.nhs.uk

Memory Clinic Information
http://www.memoryclinic.com

Age Exchange (reminiscence)
http://www.age-exchange.org.uk/

Alzheimer Solutions (information and products to help with caring)
http://www.caregiving-solutions.com

Alzheimers News
http://www.alzheimersnews.com

Latest news on Alzheimer's
http://www.alzheimerweek.org

American Health Assistance Foundation Alzheimer's Research
http://www.ahaf.org/alzdis/about/adabout.htm

Alzheimer's Caring from the Heart (practical carer information)
http://www.geocities.com/HotSprings/1159/

Alzheimer’s Disease Education and Referral Centre (ADEAR) of the US National Institute of Aging.
http://www.alzheimers.org/

Alzheimer’s: Coping with Alzheimer’s disease
http://www.geocities.com/HotSprings/3004/

NINDS Alzheimer’s information
www.ninds.nih.gov/health_and_medical/disorders/alzheimersdisease_doc.htm

Clinical trial information
http://www.veritasmedicine.com/alzheimer

Email-based support for Alzheimer carers
www.adrc.wustl.edu/alzheimer

Alzheimer's Association (USA) site for diagnosed individuals, family caregivers and friends and professionals
http://www.alz.org/

Alzheimer's Association Washington DC
http://www.alz-nca.org/

Alzheimer's Research Forum
http://www.alzforum.org/

Mayo Clinic Alzheimer’s site
http://www.mayohealth,org/home?id=3.1.2

Dementia Relief Trust (training and promoting quality care)
http://www.fordementia.org.uk

Novartis Foundation for education and innovation in healthy ageing and elderly care.
http://www.healthandage.com

Appendix XI : Books for Non-Professionals & Professionals

Personal accounts and literature

Bayley J. Iris: A Memoir of Iris Murdoch. London, Duckworth 1998. ISBN 0 7156 2848 8.

Bernlef J, Out of mind. Translated from Dutch by Adrienne Dixon . London, Faber and Faber, 1988. ISBN 0571149545

Davis R. My journey into Alzheimer's disease, Scripture Press, 1993. ISBN 1872059880

DeBaggio T. Losing My Mind: An Intimate Look at the Life with Alzheimer's.. Free Press, New York, 2002

DiEina Friel MacGowin, Living in the Labyrinth, 1993. Mainsail Press, Cambridge. ISBN 0-9518684-2-X..

Ignatieff, M, Scar tissue: a novel, Chatto and Windus, 1993. ISBN 0701141735

McGowin DF. Living in the labyrinth: a personal journey through the maze of Alzheimer's, Elder Books, 1993. ISBN 0943873185

Information for patients and carers

Alzheimer's Society. Caring for the Person with Dementia. London, Alzheimer's Society, 2002

Davidson FG. Alzheimer's: A Practical Guide for Carers to Help You Through The Day. 1994. Piatkus. ISBN 0-7499-1455-6

Cohen D, Eisdorfer C The Loss of Self: A Family Resource for the Care of Alzheimer's Disease and Related Disorders.. W.W. Norton, New York, rev. ed. 2001

Gibson HB. On The Tip of Your Tongue: Your Memory in Later Life. 1995. Third Age Press. ISBN 1-898576-05-X.

Hamdy RC, Turnbull JM, Edwards J, Lancaster MM (eds). Alzheimer's Disease: A Handbook for Caregivers. Mosby, St. Louis, 3rd ed. 1998

Mace N, Rabins PV, Castleton A, Cloke C, McEwen E. The 36-Hour Day : Caring at Home for confused elderly people, Sevenoaks, Kent, Age Concern/Hodder & Stoughton, 2nd edition, 1996.

Martyn C, Gale C. The British Medical Association family doctor guide to forgetfulness and dementia. London, Dorling Kindersley 1999. ISBN 0751306746

Murphy E. Dementia and Mental Illness in the Old. London, Papermac, 1986.

Powell LS, Courtice K . Alzheimer's Disease: A Guide for Families and Caregivers. Perseus Publishing, Cambridge, MA, 3rd ed. 2002

Sheridan C. Failure Free, Activities for the Alzheimer's Patient : a guidebook for caregivers and families. London, Macmillan, 1992.

Small D. The Memory Bible: An Innovative Strategy for Keeping Your Brain Young.. Hyperion, New York, 2002

Wilcock G. Living with Alzheimer's Disease and Similar Conditions: The Complete Self-help Guide for Family and Professional Carers. London, Penguin 1999. ISBN 0-14-0279 13X

Books for Professionals

Useful references on specific topics are listed at the end of each chapter. Some useful books on more general issues and all published in the UK or USA are listed below.

Baddeley AD, Wilson BA, Watts FN. Handbook of Memory disorders. Chichester, John Wiley & Sons, 1995.

Burns A, Howard R, Pettit W. Alzheimer's disease. A Medical Companion. Oxford, Blackwell Science, 1995. ISBN 0-632-03731-8

Burns A, Lawlor B, Craig S. Assessment scales in old age psychiatry. London, Martin Dunitz 1999 ISBN 1853175625

Burns A. Ageing and dementia: a methodological approach. London, Edward Arnold 1993. ISBN 0-340-56838-0

Cummings JL. The Neuropsychiatry of Alzheimer's disease and related Dementias. London, Martin Dunitz, 2003. ISBN 1-84184-219-2

Gauthier S. Clinical diagnoses and management of Alzheimer's disease, Second Edition. London: Martin Dunitz, 1999.
ISBN 1-85317-65-9

Goldsmith M. Hearing the Voice of People with Dementia. London, Jessica Kingsley, 1996.

Hodges JR. Cognitive Assessment for clinicians. Oxford, University Press 1994. ISBM 0-19-262395-8

Huppert FA, Brayne C, O'Connor DW. Dementia and normal ageing. Cambridge, University Press 1994. ISBN 0 521-413931.

Iliffe S, Drennan V. Primary care and Dementia. London, Jessica Kingsley Publishers, 2001. ISBN 1 85302 997 1.

Jacoby R, Oppenheimer C. Psychiatry in the Elderly, 3rd edition, Oxford, University Press 2002. ISBN 0 19 263151 9.

Jones R. Drug treatment in dementia. Oxford, Blackwell Science 2000. ISBN 0-632-05492-1.

Kitwood T. Dementia reconsidered: the person comes first. Buckingham: Open University Press, 1997. ISBN 0335198554

Kitwood T, Benson S. The New Culture of Dementia Care, London: Hawker Publications, 1995. ISBN 1874790175

Lovestone S, Gauthier S. Management of dementia. London: Martin Dunitz, 2002 ISBN 1853177393

Mulligan R, Van Der Linden M, Juillerat AC (eds). The Clinical Management of Early Alzheimer's Disease: A Handbook. Lawrence Erlbaum, Mahwah, NJ, 2002

Qizilbash N, Scheider LS, Chui H, Tariot P, Brodaty H, Kaye J, Erkinjuntti T (eds). Evidence based Dementia Practice. Oxford, Blackwell Publishing 2002. ISBN 0-632-05296-1

Rabins PV, Lyketsos CG, Steele CD. Practical Dementia Care.. Oxford: Oxford University Press, Oxford, 1999. ISBN 0-19-510625-3

Stokes G, Goudie F. (eds). The Essential Dementia Care Handbook. Bicester: Speechmark Publishing Ltd, 2002 ISBN 0863882447

Terry RD, Katzman R, Bick KL, Sisodia SS (eds) Alzheimer Disease.. Philadelphia: Lippincott, Williams and Wilkins, 1999

Wilcock G, Bucks R, Rockwood K (eds.). Diagnosis and Management of Dementia: A Manual for Memory Disorders Teams Oxford: Oxford Medical Publications, 1999
ISBN 0-19-262822-4.

Appendix XII: USEFUL ADDRESSES

International Organisations

Alzheimer's Disease International
45/46 Lower Marsh
London SE1 7RG, UK.
Phone: +44 20 7620 3011
Fax: +44 20 7401 7351
Email: info@alz.co.uk
Web: http://www.alz.co.uk

Alzheimer Europe
Route de Thionville 145
L-2611 Luxembourg
Phone: +352-297 970
Fax: +352-297 972
Email: info@alzheimer-europe.org
Web: http://www.alzheimer-europe.org/

International Psychogeriatric Association
Suite 340, 5215 Old Orchard Road
Skokie, IL 60077, USA
Phone: +1 847 663 0574
Fax: +1 847 663 0591
Email: ipa@ipa-online.org
Web: www.ipa-online.org

Help Age International
PO Box 32832
1st Floor, York House
207-221 Pentonville Road,
London N1 9UZ UK
Phone: +44 20 7278 7778
Fax: +44 20 7713 7993
Email: hai@helpage.org
Web: www.helpage.org

National Alzheimer's Disease Associations

Austria

Alzheimer Angehörige Austria
Obere Augartenstrasse 26-28
A-1020 Vienna, Austria
Phone: +43-1-332 51 66
Fax: +43-1-334 21 41
Email: alzheimeraustria@via.at
Web: http://www.alzheimer-selbsthilfe.at/

Belgium

Alzheimer Belgique a.s.b.l
Place Reine Fabiola 8
B-1083 Brussels, Belgium
Phone: +32-2-428 28 19
Fax: +32-2-428 28 19
Email: alzheimer.belgique@swing.be

Ligue Alzheimer
Clinique Le Perî,
4b Rue Montagne
Sainte Walburge
B-4000 Liège, Belgium
Phone: +32-4-225 87 93
Fax: +32-4-225 86 93
Email: henry.sabine@skynet.be
Web: http://www.alzheimer.be

Vlaamse Alzheimer Liga
Stationstraat 60-62
B-2300 Turnhout, Belgium
Phone: +32-14-43 50 60
Fax: +32-14-43 76 54
Email: vlaamsealzheimerliga@skynet.be
Web: http://www.alzheimer.be

Bulgaria

Alzheimer Bulgaria
14, Paisii Hilendarsky Str.
BG-6100 Kazanlak,
Bulgaria
Email: Nadia_Azmanova@hotmail.com

Cyprus Pancyprian Alzheimer Association
Stadiou Street 31a
CY-6020 Larnaca, Cyprus
Phone: +357-4-62 71 04
Fax: +357-4-62 71 06
Email: alzhcyprus@yahoo.com

Czech Republic Czech Alzheimer Society
Centre of Gerontology
Sˇimùnkova 1600
CZ-182 00 Praha 8, Czech Republic
Phone: +420-2-86 88 36 76
Fax: +420-2-86 88 27 88
Email: Iva.Holmerova@gerontocentrum.cz
Web: www.gerontocentrum.cz

Denmark Alzheimerforeningen
Skt. Lukas Vej 6,1
DK-2900 Hellerup, Denmark
Phone: +45-39-40 04 88
Fax: +45-39-61 66 69
Email: post@alzheimer.dk
Web: http://www.alzheimer.dk

England Alzheimer's Society
Gordon House, 10 Greencoat Place
SW1P 1PH London, U.K.
Phone: +44-20-7306 06 06
Fax: +44-20-7306 08 08
Email: enquiries@alzheimers.org.uk
Web: http://www.alzheimers.org.uk

Finland Alzheimer-keskusliitto
Luotsikatu 4 E
FIN-00160 Helsinki, Finland
Phone: +358-9-622 62 00
Fax: +358-9-62 26 20 20
Email: varpu.kettunen@alzheimer.fi
Web: http://www.alzheimer.fi

France	Association France Alzheimer 21 Boulevard Montmartre 75002 Paris, France Phone: +33 142 97 5241 Fax: +33 142 96 0470 Email: contact@francealzheimer.com Web: http://www.francealzheimer.com
Germany	Deutsche Alzheimer Gesellschaft e.V. Friedrichstr. 236 D-10969 Berlin, Germany Phone: +49-30-25 93 79 50 Fax: +49-30-31 50 57 35 Email: info@deutsche-alzheimer.de Web: http://www.deutsche-alzheimer.de
Greece	Greek Association of Alzheimer's Disease and Related Disorders Terma Dimitriou Charisi - Ano Toumba 54352 Thessaloniki, Greece Phone: +30-2310-92 58 02 Fax: +30-2310-90 90 00 Email: alzhass@med.auth.gr Web: http://www.alzheimer-hellas.gr
Hungary	Hungarian Alzheimer Society Csaba utca 7/a 1122 Budapest, Hungary Phone: +36 (1) 214 10 22 Email: ehimmer@matavnet.hu Web: http://www.tar.hu/alzheimer
Iceland	F.A.A.S. Austurbrún 31 IS-104 Reykjavík, Iceland Phone: +354-533-1088 Fax: +354-533-1086 Email: faas@alzheimer.is Web: www.alzheimer.is

Ireland	Alzheimer Society of Ireland Alzheimer House, Northumberland Avenue 43 IRL-Dúnlaoghaire. County Dublin, Ireland Phone: +353-1-284 66 16 Fax: +353-1-284 60 30 Email: info@alzheimer.ie Web: http://www.alzheimer.ie
Italy	A.I.M.A. Ripa di Porta Ticinese 21 I-20143 , Italy Phone: +39-2-89 40 62 54 Fax: +39-2-89 40 41 92 Email: aimanaz@tin.it Web: http://www.alzheimer-aima.it.
	Federazione Alzheimer Italia Via Tommaso Marino 7 I-20121 Milano. Italy Phone: +39-02-80 97 67 Fax: +39-02-87 57 81 Email: info@alzheimer.it Web: http://www.alzheimer.it
Luxembourg	Association Luxembourg Alzheimer B.P. 5021 45, rue Nicolas Hein L-1050 Luxembourg Phone: +352- 42 16 76-1 Fax: +352-42 16 76-30 Email: info@alzheimer.lu Web: http://www.alzheimer.lu
Netherlands	Stichting Alzheimer Nederland Post Bus 183 Kosterijland 3 NL-3980 CD Bunnik, Netherlands Phone: +31-30-659 69 00 Fax: +31-30-659 69 01 Email: info@alzheimer-ned.nl Web: http://www.alzheimer-ned.nl

Norway Nasjonalforeningen Demensforbundet
Oscarsgatan 36A, Postboks 7139
Majorstua, N-0307 Oslo, Norway
Phone: +47-23-12 00 00
Fax: +47-23-12 00 01
Email: post@nasjonalforeningen.no
Web: http://www.nasjonalforeningen.no

Poland Polish Alzheimer's Association
ul. Hoza 54/1
PL-00-682 Warsaw, Poland
Phone: +48-22-622 11 22
Fax: +48-22-622 11 22
Email: alzheimer_pl@poczta.onet.pl
Web: http://www.alzheimer.pl

Portugal APFADA
Av. Ceuta Norte, Quinta do Loureiro,
Lote 1 , lojas 1 e 2
1350-410 Lisboa, Portugal
Phone: +351-21-361 04 60
Fax: +351-21-361 04 69
Email: alzheimer@oninet.pt

Romania Societatea Alzheimer
Bd. Mihail Kogalniceanu 49,
sc. A et. 1 apt. 8 sector 5
RO-70603 Bucharest, Romania
Phone: +4021 334 89 40
Fax: +40722 502 239
Email: contact@alz.ro
Web: http://www.alz.ro

Scotland Alzheimer Scotland - Action on Dementia
22 Drumsheugh Gardens
EH3 7RN Edinburgh, UK
Phone: +44-131-243 14 53
Fax: +44-131-243 14 50
Email: alzheimer@alzscot.org
Web: http://www.alzscot.org

Serbia & Montenegro	Alzheimer Society of Serbia and Montenegro Dr Suhotica 6 Institute of Neurology Belgrade 11000 Serbia and Montenegro Phone: +381 11 361 4122 Fax: +381 11 684 577 Email: dpavlovic@drenik.net
Slovakia	Slovak Alzheimer Society Dubravska Str. 9 SK-842 45 Bratislava, Slovakia Phone: +421-2-63 45 26 09 Fax: +421-2-63 45 26 09 Email: alzheim@nextra.sk Web: http://www.alzheimer.sk
Spain	Alzheimer Catalunya Carrer de Còrsega 367, 2n 1a 08037 Barcelona, Spain Email: info@alzheimercatalunya.org Web: http://www.alzheimercatalunya.org/
	C.E.A.F.A. C/ Pedro Miguel Alcatarena nº 3 E-31014 Pamplona (Navarra) Spain Phone: +34-948-17 45 17 Fax: +34-948-26 57 30 Email: alzheimer@cin.es Web: http://www.ceafa.org
	Fundación Alzheimer España Pedro Muguruza 1 6c 28036 Madrid, Spain Phone: +34 91 343 11 65 Fax: +34 91 343 11 75 Email: alzheuro@yahoo.es Web: http://www.alzheimer.rediris.es

Sri Lanka Alzheimer´s and Related Disorders Foundation of Lanka
Dr.H.B.Tamitegama-President
19 Havelock Rd.
Colombo 00500
Sri Lanka
Tel.: 94 1 583 488 Fax: 94 1 732 745
E-mail alzheimers_foundation@serendib.ws

Sweden Alzheimerföreningen i Sverige
Sunnanväg 14 S Box 4109
S-222 26 Lund,
Sweden
Phone: +46-46-14 73 18
Fax: +46-46-18 89 76
Email: info@alzheimerforeningen.nu
Web: http://www.alzheimerforeningen.nu/

Demensförbundet
Drakenbergsgatan 13 nb
S-117 41 Stockholm,
Sweden
Phone: +46-8-658 52 22
Fax: +46-8-658 60 68
Email: rdr@demensforbundet.se
Web: http://www.demensforbundet.se/

Switzerland Association Alzheimer Suisse
Rue des Pêcheurs 8
CH-1400 Yverdon-les-Bains
Switzerland
Phone: +41-24-426 20 00
Fax: +41-24-426 21 67
Email: alz@bluewin.ch
Web: http://www.alz.ch

Ukraine Ukraine Association for Problems of Alzheimer's Disease
Institute of Gerontology
67 Vyshgorodskaya Street
04114 Kiev,
Ukraine
Phone: +380 44 431 0526
Fax: +380 44 432 9956
Email: bachinskaya@geront.kiev.ua

Other Patient/Carer Organisations

Down's Syndrome Association
155 Mitcham Road
Tooting
London SW17 9PG
UK
Phone: +44 20 8682 4001
Fax: +44 20 8682 4012
Email: info@downs-syndrome.org.uk
Web: http://www.dsa-uk.com/

Foundation for People with Learning Disabilities
83 Victoria Street,
London SW1H 0HW,
UK
Phone: +44 20 7802 0300
Fax: +44 20 7802 0301
Email: fpld@fpld.org.uk
Web: http://www.learningdisabilities.org.uk/

Multiple Sclerosis Society
MS National Centre
372 Edgware Road
Staples Corner
London NW2 6ND
UK
Phone: +44 20 8438 0700
Fax: +44 20 8438 0701
http://www.mssociety.org.uk

Stroke Association
240 City Road
London EC1V 2PR,
UK
Phone: +44 20 7566 0300
Fax: +44 20 7490 2686
Email: info@stroke.org.uk
Web: http://www.stroke.org.uk/

Terrence Higgins Trust (HIV & AIDS charity)
52-54 Grays Inn Road
London WC1X 8JU, UK
Phone: +44 20 7831 0330
Fax: +44 20 7242 0121
Email: info@tht.org.uk
Web: http://www.tht.org.uk/

Parkinson's Disease Society of the UK
United Scientific House
215 Vauxhall Bridge Road
London, SW1V 1EJ , UK
Phone: +44 (0)207 931 8080
Web: www.parkinsons.org.uk/

Pick's Disease Support Group
National Hospital for Neurology and Neurosurgery
8-11 Queen Square
London WC1N 3BG, UK
Web: http://www.pdsg.org.uk

Huntington's Disease Association
108 Battersea High Street
London SW11 2HT, UK
Phone: +44 (0)20 7223 7000
Web: http://www.hda.org.uk

Progressive Supranuclear Palsy (PSP-Europe) Association
The Old Rectory
Wappenham
Towcester
Northants
NN12 8SQ, UK
Phone: +44 1327 860299
Fax: +44 1327 861007
Email: psp.eur@virgin.net
Web: http://www.pspeur.org

Other Useful Contacts

Action on Elder Abuse
1268 London Road
LONDON SW16 4ER, UK
Phone: +44 20 8765 7000
Fax: +44 20 8679 4074
Email: enquiries@elderabuse.org.uk
Web: http://www.elderabuse.org.uk

Age Concern England
1268 London Road
London SW16 4ER, UK
Phone: +44 (0)800 009966
Web: www.ace.org.uk

Carers National Association
20-25 Glasshouse Yard
London, EC1A 4JT , UK
Phone: +44 (0)20 7490 8818
Web: www.carersonline.org.uk

Counsel and Care
16 Bonny Street
London NW1 9PG, UK
Phone: +44 (0)20 7485 1566
Web: www.charitynet.org/~counsel+care/

Crossroads Association
10 Regent Place
Rugby CV21 2PN, UK
Phone:+44 (0)1788 573653
Web:www.crossroads.org.uk/

Centre for Social Research on Dementia
University of Stirling
Stirling FK9 4LA, Scotland
Tel: +44 1786 466300
Fax: +44 1786 466846
Email: vag1@stir.ac.uk
Web: www.dementia.stir.ac.uk

Help the Aged
207-221 Pentonville Road
London
N1 9UZ
UK
Phone: +44 20 7278 1114
Fax: +44 20 7278 1116
Email: info@helptheaged.org.uk
Web: www.helptheaged.org.uk

Princess Royal Trust for Carers
142 Minories
London
EC3N 1LB
UK
Phone: +44 (0)20 7480 7788
Website: www.carers.org/

The Royal Association for Disability and
Rehabilitation (RADAR)
12 City Forum
250 City Road
London EC1V 8AF, UK
Phone: +44 (0)207 2503222
Website: www.radar.org.uk

Appendix XIII: DEVELOPMENTS IN DEMENTIA CARE IN THE CZECH REPUBLIC & SRI LANKA

Czech Republic

The Czech Alzheimer's Society (CAS) was founded in 1996 and recognised as a non-governmental organisation in the following year. At that time, there was little information available about Alzheimer's disease or other dementing conditions and few scientists or clinicians specialized in the area. Little attention was given to the problems of patients, their families and friends.

From the time of its formation, the CAS has focused on addressing the needs of people affected by dementia and the needs of their carers and on defending their rights and interests. A new approach to care has been promoted, with the opening of specialist day centres and provision of expert information to the public and professionals.

An early challenge was the difficult task of making available to patients the new cognitive enhancer drugs for Alzheimer's disease. The first acetylcholinesterase inhibitor, donepezil, was registered in the Czech Republic in 1998 and rivastigmine and galantamine and the glutamate antagonist memantine have followed. Pharmaceutical companies worked for them to be listed as drugs covered by health insurance, but many obstacles were placed in their path and finally the issue was only settled after the intervention of an ombudsman. The new drugs for dementia are now covered by insurance, but can only be prescribed by psychiatrists, neurologists or geriatricians who follow strict guidelines regarding diagnosis and follow up.

The CAS opened its first Day Care Centre for people with dementia in the Gerontological Institute in Prague. Patients and family members can meet there and get help and information. Patients can also be screened there for dementia and followed up by specialist physicians. Recently the CAS has developed its own database and website (www.alzheimer.cz and www.gerontologie.cz) with news, letters and questions and answers. CAS also publishes regularly the magazine "Actualities in Gerontology" (in association with the Czech Gerontological and Geriatric Society and Association of Pensioners).

There are now some 31 branches of the CAS spread throughout the Czech Republic and offering the same help and support provided by the mother organisation. A great help has been the grants offered by Phare, financed by the European Commission.

Recently, Memory Clinics have begun to open as part of departments of psychiatry and neurology, as well as those that are university-based. Regular meetings are being organised in different parts of the country and there is increasing awareness of the growing challenge of dementia.

Sri Lanka

Sri Lankans are living longer and soon will have a life expectancy equal to that of people in many developed nations.

Recent demographic information published by the Department of Census and Statisticsand corroborated b the Department of Demography of the University of Colombo indicate that life expectancy of Sri Lankans has increased between the years 1920 and 1990 by over 100% - males from 32.7 to 71.1 years and females from 30.7 to 74.8. The age structure of the population is projected to change from a pyramidal profile to a rectangular one over the next 40 years: the proportion aged under 15 years will shrink from 31% to 14%, whilst the over 60 group will expand from 8% to 28%.

The ageing syndrome is a worldwide phenomenon and Sri Lanka sits at the apex, with the dubious honour of being the country with the highest rate of ageing. This will result in an exponential increase in the number of dependant and disabled elders.

Based on international figures, it is likely that there are already many elderly Sri Lankans afflicted with dementia, perhaps 100,000 to 200,000. Demographic projections predict that this number will rise to epidemic proportions of 400,000 to 500,000. The family and social implications of this are daunting. There is a great need for accurate studies of prevalence of dementia, the nature of care-giving and the resultant burden on families and the community. This is on the future agenda of the Alzheimer's and Related Disorders Foundation of Lanka, also known as the Lanka Alzheimer's Foundation (LAF).

The LAF was incorporated formally as a private foundation on March 23rd, 2001 in cooperation and full knowledge of senior officials of Alzheimer Disease International. There were 14 people who assisted in the initiation and first year's operation. It is hoped that the Foundation will establish a solid foundation, enabling it to make contact with elders, elder groups and organisations, carers and caregivers and all other related members of the lay and professional community across the country. It is hoped that this may promote the development of requisite services for the direct welfare and happy living of the growing numbers of people affected by dementia.

INDEX

Page numbers in bold refer to a major chapter entry

Notes:

Notes:

Notes:

Notes:

Notes: